My Stroke ...
A Will to Recover

My Stroke ...
A Will to Recover

Renee Wines

iUniverse, Inc.
New York Lincoln Shanghai

My Stroke ... A Will to Recover

iUniverse books may be ordered through booksellers or by contacting:

iUniverse
2021 Pine Lake Road, Suite 100
Lincoln, NE 68512
www.iuniverse.com
1-800-Authors (1-800-288-4677)

Because of the dynamic nature of the Internet, any Web addresses or links contained in this book may have changed since publication and may no longer be valid.

The views expressed in this work are solely those of the author and do not necessarily reflect the views of the publisher, and the publisher hereby disclaims any responsibility for them.

ISBN: 978-0-595-47223-9 (pbk)
ISBN: 978-0-595-91506-4 (ebk)

Printed in the United States of America

Dedicated to ...

Mom—I want to thank you for always being supportive of everything I do, for all the times you were there for me after my many surgeries, and for being my best friend.

Kevin—Thank you for always being there for me, being a great listener, and for being the type of husband every girl dreams of having, I love you with all my heart.

CONTENTS

Acknowledgements

It is with the utmost gratitude that I thank ... Candi Sary, Mom, Lynn Coley, Stanley Sefman, and my wonderful husband, Kevin Wines.

For helping me bring this book to life.

CHAPTER 1

▼

("Be strong and
Don't lose courage,
For there is a reward
for your work.")
Chronicles 15:7

Looking back at my life, I have managed to deal with heartaches that most couldn't bear. Inspired by the strength and courage of three women in my life, my grandmother, mother, and aunt, I am the woman I am today. The memory of my grandmother on my mother's side always makes me smile because of the love we shared for each other. She was a productive woman in the working world, back in the sixties. She was a small framed woman with blond hair. She was the head bookkeeper for the Maas Brothers Company and had an excellent work ethic. She took pride in her appearance daily. She spent time primping to look her best for work and in her day to day life making sure every detail was perfect. The funniest memory I have of her is, while on a visit to her home in Florida, she picked me up after her weekly hair salon appointment where she'd had her hair styled. I was able to choose anything I wanted to do that day. I was six or seven at the time, and I chose to go swimming in the local swimming pool because of the slide in the pool. I wasn't the best swimmer so Nana promised me she would wait at the bottom of the slide to catch me when I came down. When I climbed the ladder to the top of the slide, I was so excited. I looked down at my grandmother with her freshly styled hair, and I scooted to the edge. Down the slide I went, like a huge rock plunging toward the pool. All of a sudden, I hit the water and a big wave went up in the air and down all over my Nana's freshly done hairstyle. As soon as I caught my breath, I was apologizing sincerely with every gasp for ruining her hair. Surprisingly Nana busted out with laughter, and then I started laughing, and then came tears of laughter. We were laughing so hard that we could barely walk to the edge of the pool, where we had to hold on because we were laughing so hard. Her disappointment over her ruined, freshly styled hair was overcome by the joy and love for me and how ironically funny it was. I heard Nana had battled and overcome alcoholism the next few years, before alcoholism was heard of as a huge problem. She had a will and determination to conquer where others just gave up. Every summer I spent at her home, I never noticed that she was battling the demon of alcoholism. We spent most of our time baking and making crafts together. My grandparents and I loved each other so much, we could hardly wait until each summer to see each other, and my grandfather was my biggest fan catering to my every wish. Brownie, my grandfather, and Nana would eat out at Mickies restaurant every Friday night and would save the after dinner mints all year to give to me because they knew I loved them so much. At the time Brownie was the only male figure in my life; my father was an alcoholic that chose his alcohol over me when my mother decided to leave him for a better life in Las Vegas with her twin sister. Brownie died of an aneurism a few years later while my mother, stepfather and I were on a family vacation in Mexico. I was too young to attend the funeral to say my goodbyes, so I said my goodbyes through prayers to God and asked him to take care of Brownie while in heaven and let him know I would always love him. While in high school Nana came to live with us because she had been diagnosed with terminal liver cancer, I suppose it was brought on by the alcoholism. Hospice would visit our house weekly to try and ease Nana's pain. Hospice was an organization that helped family members and their loved ones with terminal illness. Through all of Nana's pain I never once saw her cry or complain, however, I knew the pain was there when I witnessed my mother giving her pain pills hourly.

Nana stayed in the guest room of our house. I loved doing her hair and make-up, and I knew how Nana liked looking her best so I would wake up early each morning before school to fix her hair and make-up for the day. It seemed I would see a sparkle of hope behind her eyes when I would hold up a mirror for her to see herself. Despite all of my prayers, Hospice advised us to stop feeding Nana. Her body was shutting down and she could no longer eat on her own. I could not emotionally understand this and I still held out hope that Nana would overcome the cancer that invaded her body.

One night, everyone had eaten dinner except for Nana. After everyone went to bed, I snuck out to the kitchen. I opened up a can of chicken soup; Nana always told me that chicken soup could heal anything. I quietly heated the soup and tasted a little bit to make sure it wasn't too hot. I quietly walked down the hall and opened up Nana's door. I sat at the edge of her bed and set the bowl of soup on a towel on top of my lap. I scooped up the soup onto the spoon, instructed Nana to open wide, put the spoon in her mouth and I told her to try and swallow. After each bite, I would massage her throat until I thought she swallowed. I wasn't sure if Hospice was right to advise us not to feed her, and yet I was also unsure about my decision to go against their advice. So I decided to stop feeding her after a few swallows of soup, kissed her forehead, tucked her under the covers, and said goodnight. I spent most of the night praying for Nana to get better. When morning came, it was too late. My mother opened my door and yelled with emotion, "She's gone! Nana has passed away!" Half of me felt a sense of guilt for what I had done, but the other half knew that Nana would know eternally that I loved her with all of my heart. We were all grieving for the matriarch of the family; we missed the woman who showed us that one could be happy after disappointment and sadness, and that laughter lives in us all even in times of sadness. My sense to feel laughter after disappointment died that day with Nana, but her strength would live in me forever.

As a family, we collectively thought that it would be nice if I were the one to do Nana's make-up and hair for the funeral. The day before the funeral, I walked into the funeral home. I was led back to a room where Nana laid on a table. I brought all of the colored make-up to her liking and my hair utensils for styling. I was afraid because I was touching Nana's body after death but I loved her so much, I had to pull every ounce of strength I had to complete the duty I was asked to do. I started with her make-up. I touched her cold, hard face with the make-up sponge, while wiping away my tears with each stroke. I then styled her hair just the way she liked it. I felt proud that I could do this for her but just the memory of that day brings a sadness that still lives in me.

My Aunt Lynn was oozing with strength she inherited from Nana. Lynn was a beautiful, small framed woman with blond hair, chiseled features, and a turned up nose. She found a lump in her left breast during a self-examination in her bath tub. Lynn went to the doctor immediately to check out the mysterious lump; she was diagnosed with breast cancer. She was scheduled for removal of the lump. My mother and stepfather Stan were in the waiting room of the hospital when the surgeon approached them to say they were encountering a few problems and they would have to remove the whole breast. Stan felt the blood draining from his head and had to lie down because he was afraid of passing out from the news he just heard. My mother Linda comforted my stepfather until the surgery was over. The surgeon came out of the room to tell them he got all of the cancer. A sense of relief came over our whole family. One year later, Lynn found another lump, this time in her right breast. She was scheduled for a full mastectomy of her breasts, and she was sent home with drainage tubes that came out of her chest to her back. Each morning my mother would drop me off at Lynn's house to care for her for the day. I was fifteen, but I was happy to do it because I loved my aunt so much. I drained her drainage tubes twice a day to avoid infection, I wanted to do anything to make her feel comfortable and ease her pain through this. Lynn never complained and she never let anyone see the emotional strain and sadness this was putting on her self-esteem. My mother had to be very diligent about her own self breast exams. She too, was a beautiful, small framed woman with blond hair, chiseled features and a turned up nose. Just like her twin sister, Lynn. Though very thorough with her exams, my mother found a lump in her breast four years later. My mother was scheduled for a full mastectomy of both breasts to ensure no spreading would occur. Like a pattern that was instilled in our family, my mother never complained from the pain or loss of feeling under her arm. The doctor had to remove lymph nodes under her arm to make sure no cancer spread. Like my aunt, I was there for my mother. I would help wash under her arm where she couldn't feel, and help her with her exercises to regain strength after the extensive surgery. The exercises included walking the wall with her fingertips up and down like a spider crawling. I could see her pain through her facial squinting but never once did I hear any complaining. She wasn't happy to be without her womanly pride, having lost both of her breasts, but she showed bravery with the circumstances that were dealt to her. My stepfather never let on that he saw her as any less of a woman. His love for her was stronger than ever and even more, given the incredible strength she showed. These events would set the tone for my life—bravery, courage, and strength in the midst of tragedy and illness.

CHAPTER 2

▼

("Always in every prayer
Of mine for you, all
Making request with joy")
Philippians 1:4

I lived the Las Vegas lifestyle. There was always excitement and I was always on the go. As a teenager I hung around with upper class kids from the wealthiest of families, though my family was just middle class. My parents continually struggled to hold businesses together—car dealerships and clothing stores. My uncle advised my step-dad to get into the clothing business as he had made a fortune off them, himself. They never made it big, but they were successful enough to provide my family with a beautiful four bedroom home in an upscale neighborhood and sports cars to our liking. My parents gave me everything they could, but they could never give me the kinds of things that my wealthier friends had. The relationship I had with my parents was much different than that of my wealthier friends. Our relationship was based on love instead of material things. I had a relationship with the same boyfriend all through high school and the years following. Danny was from Uruguay, South America. He had tan skin, baby blue eyes, and chiseled features. I started a relationship with him because he was the most popular guy in high school and the best looking. Once we were together he made me feel as though he were doing me a favor, just to be with me. After all, he could have any one, he said. To him, in his words, I was a gringo. I broke up with him once and he begged me to get back with him for a week. I went back just so I didn't have to hear it anymore.

I had no direction in life after high school but my mom noticed a given talent I had in hairstyling. She always asked me to do her hair because she couldn't do it like I could. She noticed I was at my happiest while doing hair. My mom came home one day to let me know she enrolled me into beauty school. I wanted to make my parents proud so I agreed to go. My mother saw a love I hadn't even see. I ended up completing 1800 hours of beauty school and received A's on all of my tests. I still kept up my week-end lifestyle of going out with my friends but made sure I was promptly at beauty school on Monday morning. I went to school with my best friend from high school, Gina. She took the manicurist classes. After graduating from beauty school, we went from shop to shop together. I worked very hard on building my clientele. Word of mouth was my main source of building. I kept up on all the latest haircut fashions, coloring, and perm-ing. My specialty was spiral perming. All of my co-workers would refer their spiral perms to me because I was the only one who would have enough patience to sit and roll hair for four hours at a time, plus these perms would bring in $150.00 a job. I would have clients from California fly in just so I could cut and color their hair. My bulk clientele were men: business owners, contractors, salesmen, casino poker dealers, and most of the men hairstylists I worked with. I was told that men preferred me because of my skill, my looks, and my easygoing personality. Things seemed to be going well, I enjoyed my job, and I enrolled in all the latest hair coloring classes to stay current. Danny asked me to move in with him. He had purchased a fixer upper duplex that he gutted out. Together we made all of the remodeling decisions along with picking out the furniture. Danny always said that the house was ours, but I felt like a visitor. He wanted to make sure I knew he was the one who worked hard to purchase the house and had enough money to buy the furniture. Because of his arrogance and controlling personality, my feelings for him started to change. It seemed like I spent most of my time at home cleaning the house. I was already a very neat person, but sharing a home with Danny presented a new challenge—cleaning *his* way. I had to squeegee down the shower doors without missing a spot, I had to vacuum and get the lines just right, and when I made the bed the folds were expected to be perfectly tucked under. I only agreed to his every command because I would rather do it than hear his ranting and raving if I didn't. His expectations in the kitchen were even more difficult than the housecleaning. Danny expected a four course dinner on the table every night. Needless to say, we ate take-out a lot. He would rather eat somewhere else than wait until I got everything on the table without meeting his standards. Danny's temper could fly out of control if I didn't watch it, just as it did on a vacation to California once. He didn't like my outfit, but I told him I liked the way I looked. The next thing I knew and felt was an opened hand slap across my face, this happened in front of a crowd at a night club. I felt stunned and dizzy as I almost fell to the ground. I got back to the hotel, and my face stayed red for the rest of the night. Danny would always make me feel less than a woman to his family. I wanted to be a wife, this was in my blood. I knew I could be a good wife under different circumstances.

I was so frustrated and disgusted with him at this point, I didn't even want him to touch me. Within my group of friends and social groups I heard of a very well-known, good looking man who had interest in me. I knew of Steve but never thought he'd look twice at me because he was so successful and my self-esteem was so depleted from dealing with Danny. I was so excited and flattered. I felt this was a way to get out of a bad relationship. I hired a trainer to help me with working out so I could spend as little time at home as possible. All of my friends were into working out and I wanted to make sure I looked good as a way to meet some one else. The Hard Rock Café was the popular hang out for Vegas kids. My friends and I spent a lot of weekends there. I was always the one that ended the night in control of my surroundings and the reliable designated driver who drove my sloppy drunk friends home safely. One night while I was enjoying my one beer at the bar, my friends came running up to me. They were so excited to let me know Steve wanted to talk to me and was coming my way. He sat on the stool next to me. My palms got clammy and my heart was racing. I was in awe of his good looks, blue eyes, and dark hair. His success was just the icing on the cake. Steve's attention lay on every word I said. His eyes never looked away from mine once. I was so happy to have so much positive attention. I let him know right away that I had a boyfriend as he put his business card in my hand. He had a confidence about him. The smile didn't leave my face the rest of the night. The drive home that night was never ending. I didn't want to go home. I loved the weekend outings with my friends because I was away from Danny. I thought I loved him but I was just staying because I was a creature of habit. I didn't know how to get out of it. I talked to my mother over the phone every day during this time. She and my step-dad had moved out to California to start a car dealership just after I graduated from beauty school. After my mom had battled with breast cancer and had a full mastectomy just before she left, she had to take numerous pain pills to counteract the pain. The amount she was taking far exceeded the prescribed recommended dose. While in California her addiction spun out of control. As busy as I was, my thoughts and worry over my mother never drifted far from my mind. She longed for the company of her twin and me. My step-dad was working seven days a week to keep the new business afloat. My mother's loneliness caused her to leave him and move back to Las Vegas to be closer to me and live with her twin. I felt stuck in a relationship I was miserable in. My business wasn't bringing in enough money to afford my rent for my chair at the salon and rent for an apartment of my own, so I could leave him. I chose to continue my relationship with someone I didn't love for the sake of having a roof over my head, but I still wanted to find love, even if it meant being unfaithful to Danny. I'd had Steve's business card in my wallet for a week. On Friday I gave into temptation and called his cell phone. We would meet at The Hard Rock at 9:00PM. I walked into the Hard Rock and Steve was already there waiting for me. Our eyes caught each other as we both smiled. The physical attraction was so strong; we were drawn to each other. We continued to see each other each weekend. He would call me at work three to four times a day. He started dropping off gifts to me at my work—leather boots, Rolex watch, tennis bracelet, belts, etc. I was falling in love with this man, five years my senior. Danny would continue to pick me apart daily, and belittle me. I quietly put up with him knowing that the weekend would soon come and I'd get to be with Steve again. On one hand I felt a sense of guilt for my indiscretions. On the other hand, I wasn't married and Danny treated me like a doormat anyway. The Las Vegas lifestyle was in full swing each weekend, when I was introduced to two brothers new in town, George and Gavin. Gavin was dating a friend of mine. They were in town to build a new casino called The Palms. I didn't think much of it. The trust I had for what men told me was gone. George invited me to go to the governor's ball, I could sense his kind heart and how powerful he was. I accepted. I arrived at George's mansion and everywhere I looked I saw fresh flowers. He had them flown in daily just for the smell. I felt like a princess when we drove to the ball in his brand new red Mercedes. The dinner was served in formal settings. I saw George one other time after that first date at the ball, but my heart was with Steve. George was too busy opening up his casino. I would arrive every other day to meet my trainer. She was impressed with my energy and determination to get my body into shape. Afterwards I would drive across the street to my job. I arrived early and I would leave late. I was booking full days, back to back clients. Danny wanted me to be on birth control pills to avoid unwanted pregnancies. He wanted me to make an appointment with Planned Parenthood to get a prescription for birth control pills. I didn't want any unwanted pregnancies either so I agreed. I didn't know of the dangers of birth control except for what they said on the back of the package: May cause high blood pressure and stroke. I had no reason to worry; only cancer ran in my family. I had to have monthly appointments with Planned Parenthood to check blood pressure and to do routine papsmears. For months, my papsmear came back negative. One month, it came back class 2 with high blood pressure. Planned Parenthood referred me to gynecologist Dr. Redding. She reviewed my original test from Planned Parenthood and took some tests of her own. She informed me I was in the beginning stages of cervical cancer. They were small lesions in growth. She also noted that my blood pressure was extremely high. She had to take me off of the birth control pills. I felt my heart drop because I knew Danny wouldn't be with me if I wasn't on birth control pills. I still wasn't making quite enough money to live on my own. I had been seeing Steve for six months when I heard he was married with two children. I let him know that we should break it off. He began frantically explaining why he had to lie about his wife; he was in love with me from day one. He was holding one of his newly built homes for me. The condition for the home was I had to break it off with Danny. I felt secure that Steve had a place for me, so letting Danny know I was now off of birth control pills wasn't so bad. Once a week I would go to Dr. Redding's office to let her freeze off my lesions of cancer. On the fourth week she told me that my blood pressure had come down to normal levels. 120/80. I could get back on birth control pills again. I told Steve I was now ready to break it off with Danny, but the house he was saving had been sold; he couldn't leave his wife because she would take all of his money, and he said she probably was seeing someone on the side too. Steve invited me to go to Cabo san Lucus, Mexico with another couple. It would be a chance for us to be alone and celebrate my twenty-seventh birthday. I told Danny I was going to see my parents in California. I was expecting a romantic getaway with Steve but his attitude was, now that he had me, he could do whatever he wanted. The whole trip Steve just ignored me and spent most of his time with his pals. I couldn't wait to get back home to Las Vegas. I never wanted to see Steve again. My self-esteem was gone; I didn't feel I could trust any man. As I drove home to Danny, I had no idea what I was going to do. I walked into my home and Danny had two toy poodles in a box waiting for me as a birthday gift. The two were sisters, black and apricot in color. I named them Ginger and Stormy. Danny had always bought me gifts for the material fact. He knew how badly he treated me but wanted to show everyone else what a great guy he was. His ego needed that. Still, I was so happy because I was still in mourning over my poodle Amber that I adored. She got out and was run over by a car a couple months previous. I didn't believe Amber was dead until I held her bloodied body covered in a blood soaked towel. Her heart was on the outside of her chest. A month before Amber's death I was mourning over the death of a co-worker. Cynthia and I were like sisters. We hit it off because of the similar drive we had to do hair. Cynthia was the most popular hairstylist in the salon; her biggest client was Andre Agassi. We ate lunches together, shopped together, discussed hair and products together. She was afraid for her life when she ran off to Arizona. Her abusive boyfriend wanted to kill her. On this trip she was hit broadside by a mail truck. She was wearing a seatbelt but was hit so hard that her brain stem was shaken too much to survive the impact. With Cynthia's death, my mom's addiction, my uncle's recent suicide over having Aids, Steve, Danny, I was feeling emotionally strained over so many people that I loved. One night after work, I was home talking on the phone to a good friend. I started having severe stomach cramps. I had just gotten over my menstrual cycle about two weeks prior. I've heard of severe cramping and gushing blood before miscarriage. I just blurted out to my friend, "I think I'm having a miscarriage, I better go," as I hung up the phone. I went and sat on the toilet. A quarter-size dropping of mass dropped out of me. The blood was running out of me like a raging river. I stood in the shower to see if that helped but there was so much blood I started feeling dizzy. I called Danny home from work. I put the mass into a plastic sandwich baggy to take to Dr. Redding. She tested the mass. It came back as a six week old fetus. I had no idea I was pregnant. A gut feeling told me I was when the cramping started. The Friday and Saturday ritual outing came and went. Sunday came, my head started to hurt on the right side over my ear. I didn't think much of it, I never had headaches. I figured I was getting a cold. I started taking Dayquil cold medicine. That always helped me when I was sick in the past. Monday came, the headache from the day before was still with me. I thought *this cold is going to be bad when it gets here*. I had to take Dayquil plus aspirin just to help me get through the day, because the pain had escalated in strength. Monday night my head still hurt. Tuesday morning I awoke with the pain that was now becoming too familiar. I had to hurry because my books were full with clients every hour. I had to meet up with my trainer before work too. I wanted to look pretty that day because my naturally curly hair attracted new clients. I threw the Dayquil in my purse and ran out the door. I worked out really hard at the gym; the headache, oddly, seemed to subside a little bit. As I walked into work, I felt such a sense of extreme happiness to be going to work. I loved making people look pretty. This was the only place I felt secure and proud to be me.

CHAPTER 3

▼

(Though I walk through the valley of the
Shadow of death,
I will fear no evil,
For thou art
with me)
Psalms 23:4

4:00PM, 5/3/97: My headache exploded in my brain above my right ear, and after the third day, it almost seemed as though this pain had become a part of me. I just finished my last client's haircut when the pain seemed to intensify. I had to find a way to rid myself of this pain. I asked my friend if I could have an ibuprofen that she used for her menstrual cramps. After taking this, by the time I walked back to my work station, I looked into the mirror. The pain escalated in strength with a sudden feeling of numbness. My face fell from lack of muscle tone on the left side. The room began to spin as terror filled my body. My friend ran to my aid along with others. I couldn't hold myself up. The weight of my left side made it impossible for me to stand. The lack of muscle tone extended my whole left side. I collapsed. "Call 911," I heard many say. I said, "No, I'm just having an allergic reaction to the pill I just took." I fell into semi-consciousness. I could hear and feel the paramedics working effortlessly on me. However, I didn't have the cognitive ability to recognize exactly what was happening to me. In the ambulance, the paramedics were asking trivial questions as to get a better understanding of how my brain was working. "Who is our president?" "What is today's date?" I answered all of their questions with accuracy. I felt the ambulance speed up each time my blood pressure and heart rate was taken. I could hear the ambulance siren. It was almost as if I was in a fog, everything seemed gray in color. I was looking at my life playing in a black and white film in slow motion. I was rushed to the Valley Hospital trauma unit. It was there that I was assigned a neurologist. He later determined that I had suffered a massive stroke. My friends and family were in the waiting room confused as to why and how this could have happened, I was a twenty-seven-year-old healthy woman. In my hospital bed the film was still rolling in black white, and slow motion. My cognitive ability still wouldn't allow me to fully understand what was going on. I was only allowed one visitor at a time—Danny followed by my mother, then my aunt. Each time they left the room, my blood pressure would rise. The pain was escalating with each passing minute. It felt as though my brain was trying to fit through my right ear canal and every tooth on the right side was decayed with cavity. In the waiting room, almost every chair was taken with a friend or family member of mine. They started a prayer chain that would continue the whole day through. I was taken for a CAT scan every thirty minutes to determine the rate of swelling due to the extreme amounts of blood surrounding my brain. When a closed head injury occurs, a person gets combative from the lack of understanding. The doctors and nurses had to tape my head down just to take the CAT scan. Dr. Lamacusa had composed himself enough to walk out and tell my mother and father who later arrived from California. They were police escorted in by Metro. A cop pulled them over for speeding. He recognized the last name and questioned the urgency. He had been a friend of mine when I took some classes at UNLV. Dr. Lamacusa had to tell them their one and only daughter only had a fifty/fifty chance to live that night. Across the town at the other hospital in Las Vegas, my uncle was admitted because of complications do to Aids. The doctor wanted to try a new medication to slow down the swelling in my brain. In the meantime, a pastor was to be called in to read my last rights. The pain had taken over the right side of my brain, I still was unaware of the extreme danger my life was in. I couldn't understand why I was in the hospital when I could move my right side with no problems. I was taken down for an angiogram so Dr. Lamacusa could see what veins were actually working. The nurses taped my head once again as terror filled my body. They inserted the dye by needle into my arm. Within seconds my head and neck felt like a fire was racing through it, I cried out in pain. The angiogram showed that the blood had destroyed all life of neurons on the right side. When a stroke occurs on one side, it's always the opposite side that becomes paralyzed. I was taken back to the trauma unit. My mom was waiting for my arrival. The lack of muscle tone to the left side of my face and cognitive ability, made forming words to speak impossible. The only thing I was able to do and understand was to form tears so my mother would get help for me. Morphine was given to numb the extreme pain I was suffering. The medication only seemed to last seconds when another explosion of pain would hit my nervous system. Danny was trying to control everyone from the nurses to anyone involved with my case. Dr. Lamacusa approached him and asked, "Does your girlfriend do any kind of drugs?" "No," he replied. "What does she do?" "She takes Ortho-Novum birth control pills," he told the doctor. "That's what caused this." Dr. Lamacusa looked relieved that he finally figured out this mystery. The angiogram showed a birth defect slow flow artery on my right side. My girlfriend who had given me the ibuprofen finally arrived at the hospital in tears. She cried out, "Did the pill I gave her, do this?" Dr. Lamacusa replied "No, you probably saved your friends life; the pill calmed her enough to be able to go through such a massive stroke." While in my hospital bed I noticed someone put her head through the curtain that surrounded my bed. A grey fog surrounded her long black hair that fell against my blanket. It was my girlfriend Cynthia. She said calmly, "Don't worry, I'm right here." I felt an immediate peace come over me. Within seconds she disappeared. Cynthia was a friend of mine who had died three months before.

Valley Hospital, Intensive Care Unit: I awoke to a whole new world I never knew existed, with Physical, Occupational, and Speech therapy. I had been in a semi—conscious state when I was downgraded from critical care to intensive care. Mr. Rutherford was the first of many physical therapists I would have. The fog that still invaded my head wouldn't allow me to understand exactly why I was in the hospital. My right side was the only thing that existed. My head only looked towards the right; my right eye was the only one working. My left peripheral vision was now blind. My face hung from lack of muscle tone on the left. My cognitive ability would not allow me to understand that I could no longer use my left arm or leg. I was now paralyzed on my left side, as if someone had drawn an invisible line down the middle of my body. Mr. Rutherford attached two electrodes to my left leg quadriceps muscle. Electrical stimulation is a machine that sends a message to the muscle to help it remember how to work. My leg did not respond because I felt nothing. I had to be monitored each time I ate any food, my tongue and throat muscles that make eating possible were also paralyzed. Each time I would eat, half of the food would fall out of my mouth onto my blanket. In between meals you could see drool from the left side of my mouth. This is known as dysphasia. This problem can range from mild drooling to severe coughing and choking. During all of this, I felt peace. I felt the presence of God, at this re-birth of the new me. The same as he was, at my birth as a child. A month would go by; to me it seemed like only days. On a daily basis I was visited by family and friends in between physical, occupational, and speech therapy. I cognitively could not understand why I kept having therapy for my left side and for my speech. I felt fine. That's how the fog worked. Inside I felt fine but everyone around me could see I was not mentally thinking clearly. One evening I felt the urge to urinate. I put my right leg over the edge of the bed while I guided my left leg off with my right hand. I stood for a moment then collapsed to the floor. I hit my head on the night table. Two nurses rushed to my aid. They yelled, "What are you doing?" "I have to go to the bathroom," I replied. "You are paralyzed and cannot walk. You have had a stroke." I was put back into my hospital bed. I was confused. *What is a stroke?* I asked myself. This was the first time anyone had told me of this. My therapists instructed Danny and my family to bring in my favorite pictures. They had to put them on my table on the left side. Each time they were to visit, they had to stand on my left side. The therapists wanted me to start remembering that I had a left side. I had what they called left sided neglect.

On the day I was to leave Mr. Rutherford came in to say goodbye. He admired an angel figurine sitting on my table. "You can have it," I said.

"You walk back in here and give it to me," he replied. That phrase was to be one of the driving forces to walk again. I would take the figurine home with me and work my hardest to learn how to walk again just to give it to him. I was relieved and excited to be going home when the nurses wheeled me into a waiting ambulance, the fog I had was still upon me. I couldn't understand where I was going when I was driven to another hospital—Sunrise Hospital.

A stroke, also known as cerebrovascular accident (CVA), is a neurological injury where blood supply to a part of the brain has been interrupted, by a clot in the artery or an artery bursts. As a result that part of the brain dies (becomes necrotic). Strokes can be classified into two categories.

Ischemic—occur in 80–90% of strokes, a blood vessel becomes clotted and the blood supply to part of the brain is blocked.

Hemorrhagic—A hemorrhage. This occurs when a blood vessel in the brain ruptures or bleeds. Hemorrhagic strokes interrupt the brains blood supply because the bleeding vessel can't carry its blood to designated tissue. The blood irritates brain tissue, disrupting the chemical balance, causing intracranial pressure restricting blood flow to brain tissue. Hemorrhagic strokes are the more dangerous of the two strokes, I had a hemorrhagic stroke.

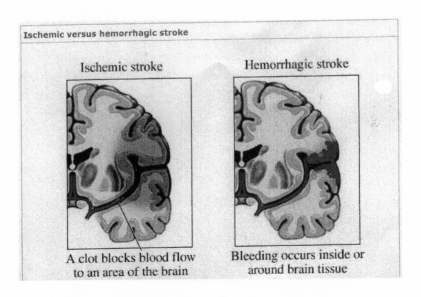

Ischemic versus hemorrhagic stroke

Ischemic stroke | Hemorrhagic stroke

A clot blocks blood flow to an area of the brain | Bleeding occurs inside or around brain tissue

Sunrise Hospital, rehabilitation unit: The third floor rehabilitation unit is where I would reside for the next six weeks. I awoke to a wheelchair sitting beside my bed. This was now to become a part of me and my way of existence. I thought to myself, "Was this really happening to me?" Two nurse's aids approached my room to say they were there to help me with ADL's. They skipped over the part about telling me what ADL's were. They started changing my hospital gown into clothes brought from home. When I looked down, at one point I was totally nude. Modesty was something I had to ignore. I felt like a rag doll a little girl was changing for the hundredth time. I later learned that ADL's were short for adult dressing lessons. For two days I had help from the aids on getting dressed. On the third, the aids came; they threw my clothes at me. "Get dressed," they said, and left my room with out saying another word. I was frustrated at first; I knew this wasn't the time to feel pity. It took me an hour to figure out how to put everything on but I did it. I still needed help with my shoes and tying the shoestrings. A nurse later wheeled me to the hallway in front of the nurse's station. A big board sat on the wall with patients' names. I could see my name in eight time slots with different therapists; I would have to look at this board daily as a map for what I would be doing each day. I was wheeled into the eating area for breakfast. The fog was still upon me but starting to clear. Everywhere I looked someone was in a wheelchair. Their ages ranged from sixty to eighty. Here I sat at age twenty-seven. I was so happy to be eating. This was a normalcy that I remember enjoying. Rice Crispies, milk, and a banana sat in front of me. My left arm lay heavily on my lap. I couldn't open the box to the Rice Crispies, the milk, or the banana. This was a first of many realizations I would have. A nurse came to my aid to help me open up everything. This was the best meal I had tasted in a long time. All of a sudden a nurse shoved her finger into my mouth, felt around the bottom and top part of the left side of my mouth. She yelled out to another nurse, "She's packin' food." Packin' food is what happens when your tongue is paralyzed and it cannot move food from inside your cheeks. A person can choke on food that is still left inside of his/her mouth. I felt violated and humiliated when my space was invaded. It seemed to me that just because I had a brain injury, they assumed I didn't know right from wrong, I felt dirty. I just wanted to take a shower and wash myself from head to toe. The only problem, I was in a wheelchair and paralyzed. I no longer knew how to take a shower on my own or wash myself from head to toe. A state of depression waved over me like blanket. At the same time strength came over me. *I have got to figure out a way to get myself well and out of here.* Each hour of every day I spent relearning how to reuse my left side. In speech therapy I would spend time reading and writing. I learned that I could not read anything on the left side of the page. I read from the middle of the sentence on. I wrote like a fifth grader, and I could not remember to cross my t's or dot my i's. It's a condition I still struggle with today. In occupational therapy, I learned that my arm was now flacid; no muscles tone whatsoever. My shoulder was subluxed. This is a condition where the collarbone separates from the muscle there is no tone to hold the bone in place. In physical therapy I met physical therapist, Bernie. He looked to be about my same age, wore thick rimmed glasses, his hair was long and hung over one eye. He looked like a computer geek. The radio was playing loudly. It was my favorite band, Depeche Mode. "How is this guy going to help me?" I thought. With my right foot, I wheeled myself into the therapy room. Bernie gave me my first lesson in wheelchair survival. "Always lock your chair." That word **your** rang out to me. Bernie helped me out of my wheelchair. He sat me on the therapy mat in front of him. He asked where I thought my left hand was. I didn't know. He said, "You are sitting on it." From then on I was to always be aware of where my left hand was. My leg was termed flacid. I was feeling some doubt about my recovery. I looked up from the mat at Bernie. I never saw a person look so confident; I felt he knew exactly what his plan of action would be for my care. My day of therapy would end at 4:30pm. I spent the rest of the early evening studying and reading the physiology of strokes from books I had brought in from friends or that I asked for from the doctor's library. If I knew exactly what happened inside my brain, I could better help myself physically get better. In my hospital bed each night I made a routine of doing sit-ups to help with core strength. I was aware of this because of my workouts with my trainer. Core muscles are what make walking and standing possible after stroke. The occupational therapists used electrical stimulation on my facial muscles to stop the drooping and paralysis. I would feel a tingling feeling, my left eye would wink, and my cheek would bounce up and down. Within only a matter of weeks, my face regained its muscle tone, however, I still would have to live with dysphasia, mild drooling. Bernie also used electrical stimulation as a source of how to get muscle tone back. For weeks I would have to lay on the mat with electrodes connected to my quadriceps. I could now feel a tingling sensation but I could not move. Every time I felt the tingling, Bernie would lift my leg in an upwards motion. My leg felt like it weighed a thousand pounds. I had to use my mind, to think of my leg moving upwards. I was fitted for an ankle brace. After each session of electrical stimuli, Bernie would lift me to the silver bars made for walking and standing. My foot moved. Bernie was so excited. He said I took a step, but I only saw my foot move millimeters. The depression weighed heavily on me. For days my left foot moved millimeters that were now known as steps. I was a perfectionist; I wanted to take a step just like the ones I used to take. Every other night Danny, along with my friends and family came to visit. I enjoyed the company but looked forward to the cards Danny would bring from friends or clients from the salon. One of the cards from my client read as follows ...

I heard you were making wonderful progress,
I know with your strength, determination, and the love of your family
and friends, you will get better.
You will always be etched in my mind as one of the most beautiful
women I have ever known.
Hang tough girl,
Carol

The space on my wall was limited where he taped them. The support was great. It drove me to want to succeed. Every Thursday was shower night. I dreaded this time the most. All of the nerves on my left side were hypersensitive from the brain injury. My nerves would overreact to anything hot or cold. A nurse's aid always helped with patients on shower nights. I had to learn to be comfortable with a stranger washing me. The water would sting my skin like fire or ice, depending on the temperature. The shower chair I sat in was hard and freezing. On one occasion a male aide was to help me, I never felt so uncomfortable. He undressed me, and I sat nude in front of him as he took the soap and washcloth to wash my body. I tried to shield myself with my right arm to the best of my ability. Once again I felt humiliated and violated. Each night before bed I prayed myself to sleep. A nurse routinely came in to put a brace on my foot to prevent drop-foot, a condition of dropping the foot due to weakness or paralysis of the foot muscles. A brace was also placed on my hand to prevent spasticity or hypertonicity, a condition in which certain muscles are continuously contracting. Contraction causes stiffness and tightness of the muscles that may interfere with movement. While I was in the hospital, Danny and I celebrated our eleventh year of dating each other. I was so thrilled when he surprised me one night. He brought all of his family. They each made a different dish for dinner. Lasagna was the main course. He popped out a small ring box out from under his clothing. I opened the box and saw a beautiful gold ring with a diamond on top. Danny proposed to me in front of his whole family. I reluctantly accepted. The feeling I had was that his proposal was more for looks instead of true love. He wanted praise as a brave person for proposing to his paralyzed girlfriend. Instead of celebrating our love, his family was celebrating by praising him. Bernie continued the use of electrical stimulation on my quadriceps muscle. We saw no effects from this, up until the day of my discharge. He connected the electrodes to my quadriceps. I felt the urge to raise my leg by will, my leg suddenly lifted. Bernie was surprised. The machine wasn't turned on yet. I was concerned that the main focus of therapy wasn't on my arm. I kept inquiring about this in the occupational department. My arm hung down by my side like a wet noodle. I needed the use of both arms to continue in my career. The day of my discharge came. Danny came to pick me up to go home. Along with paralysis, I took home with me hope, fear, anxiety, frustration, anger, sadness, and a sense of grief for my physical and mental loss.

CHAPTER 4

▼

(Pride leads to disgrace,
With humility comes wisdom)
Proverbs 11:2

I had to learn car transfers before I could leave the hospital. The occupational therapist wheeled me down to the lobby doors that lead outside. The passenger side door was open to Danny's car; she wheeled me to the passenger side. She extended a straight board from my wheelchair to the passenger seat of the car. I had to scoot my butt onto the board. She instructed me to pull my body's weight across the board towards the left into the car. It took a few practices. The dead weight of my left side made this task seem unbearable; I used my right hand and my waist to pull my weight into the car. I just wanted to go home. I wanted to get back to the life I had before the stroke. I wanted to see my dogs, Ginger and Stormy. Once I mastered car transfers, we were on the road towards home. I was unsure how I was going to carry on with my life. I still hadn't come to the reality that I just lost the career I studied so hard for, and loved so much. Danny was obsessed about how I was going to get back to the girl I once was. I obsessed about getting back to work to pick up where I left off. My clients needed me. The fog wouldn't let me see things as they were. I didn't realize how much damage the stroke did. Everything I couldn't do because of the paralysis. Reality was I had 5% of my leg working at a weakened state, and my balance was severely impaired. I couldn't find the middle for equilibrium. Every time I stood up, my body leaned to the right. This felt normal to me. Normal weight bearing consisted of weight evenly distributed to both the right and left legs. In my brain, my middle consisted only of the right side of my body. The brain damage has made me neglect to feel my left side completely. My arm felt like a thousand pound wet noodle hanging by my side. Danny had arranged for nurses and home therapy three times a week. We were disappointed to find out Bernie did not work for home therapy, we had confidence in him. He was the only one who made my muscles respond to treatment. Danny made it clear that I had to get my body back to 100% full use. I was happy that Danny was really going to go the extra mile with me and my disabilities but it soon became clear it was all for looks and his ego. He wanted me to be the model he first started dating. Reality was I couldn't be that just then. He had ramps built onto the front and back steps that lead into the house. Danny approached Bernie with an offer to pay him under the table while treating me. He would come to my home after his job at the hospital. Bernie accepted. I was fitted with an orthotic. It was a hard, plastic brace. By day I would wear a brace for my ankle, by night I wore a brace for my hand. We had to stay one step ahead of the spasticity. The orthotic brace helped to stabilize the ankle while standing or walking. I saw Bernie twice a week. He concentrated on getting my core muscles stronger and helping me to find my middle. I had a home exercise routine plan plus therapists all through the week. Danny made a chart of times, exercise routines, and repetitions of the exercises I had to do. He always made a point of telling me I had to be 100%. He wouldn't accept anything less. Danny would call every thirty minutes from his glass shop. It was a business he started at age twenty-five; it did well in the Las Vegas area. He wanted to make sure I was doing the exercises he laid out for me; he treated me like an employee. He was in control of every aspect of my life. I never would have imagined how controlling he would become. Feeling tired or having overworked muscles wasn't acceptable to him. Therapy was the only thing I was able to think about. The home occupational therapist was treating me three times a week. I worried about how I would ever work again. Reality is I would never cut hair again. I was now getting income from the state, Social Security Income. I was paid a little over $300.00 a month. The nurses came every other day to help with my showers. Taking a shower was still an unpleasant experience. I still had to use a hard, cold shower chair to sit in while taking a shower. The hypersensitivity still stung like fire or ice, depending on the temperature of the water. On one occasion, a nurse was so over-weight, I estimated by at least 200 pounds, that sweat was rolling down her face. Every time she overexerted herself to wash my body, she made the sound of a dog panting. I couldn't wait until it was over. I was tired of people touching me or probing me. She was there to help me but I was so afraid she was going to pass out on me. I was only 110 pounds. How would I help her? I was paralyzed. I was sitting in the shower on the shower chair, naked. I didn't see my wheelchair anywhere. I had no way of getting to a phone to call 911. We hurried through my shower so the nurse could finally rest by sitting on my couch. I quickly learned that the insurance company I was contracted with was controlling every part of my therapy. About three weeks before my stroke happened, I wasn't able to afford to pay the premium on my insurance. My business was slow at the time. Danny paid the premium for me. I was confident to take their physical. I never took street drugs and I hardly drank alcohol. I had no pre-existing illnesses. The day I had the stroke was the day Danny's check went through the bank. Danny wanted to control everything. He wouldn't even let me open any of my own mail. Each time I had to use the bathroom, I had to tell him where I was going. His mentality was that I had a brain injury. He made me feel I couldn't do anything without him. He was treating me the same as the nurses did in the hospital. I wondered where that caring person went; the person that was so interested in helping me in the hospital, the one who rented movies for us to watch, my favorite movie was "The other side of the mountain", the true story of the professional skier that skied off the mountain and was paralyzed from the neck down. Where was the man who engaged me? I wasn't even married yet and I was miserable. Danny was a perfectionist to a fault. His fiancé wasn't perfect anymore. I couldn't use my left side anymore; I was like a child he didn't want. I wasn't the trophy girl I once was. This was taken away from him in a split second just as my world was taken from me. Two letters came from the insurance company. The first letter informed us that they felt I had enough therapy. I grew concerned while most of my left side still lay flacid. The letter said I should be well by now. I knew a month of hospital therapy and four weeks of home occupational therapy wasn't going to bring back muscle tone after a massive stroke. Through my reading, I learned every stroke is different in the way one heals depending on which part of the brain it hits. My stroke mostly affected my motor skills. All home therapy was cut off. The depression I felt weighed heavily on my shoulders. "How can I get well without therapy?" I had to fight to get well. I had to stay strong and work harder. The second letter read that they were denying all payments to the trauma unit and to the rehabilitation hospitals. It said that the stroke must have been pre-exiting. They had the right to deny payment. All of my payments to the insurance company were paid on time. I passed their initial physical. Bernie came every Tuesday and Thursday. Payments to him were not coming from the insurance company. I couldn't believe the insurance company was trying to get out of a $30,000 bill. I was angered at the unfairness. I contacted the newspaper and channel 8 news. Channel 8 news wanted the story. The subject was how unfair insurance companies were, stroke, and the dangers of birth control pills for young women. Danny informed the insurance appeals department that we were taking our complaint to the channel 8 news center. A few days later, I received a third letter from the insurance company. I wasn't allowed to open the letter addressed to me. Danny treated me as a brain dead vegetable. Reality was, my stroke mostly affected my movement. He was now paying all the bills and loved the control he had over the situation. The letter from the insurance company stated that they were paying the bill in full. Danny worked twelve hours a day at his glass shop. He would go out to the night clubs every Friday and Saturday until all hours of the morning, something I used to do. I was left alone most of the time. He carried on as if I never had a stroke. As his fiancé, I felt more like a bother than a loved one. I couldn't help but feel my heart crying invisible tears. The visits from my girlfriends became fewer and farther apart until I had no visits. I only got an occasional call once in a while. I noticed things had changed inside my body since the stroke. My left side had extreme hypersensitivity. To brush my hair was extremely painful, the knots in my hair started building up. I could barely touch my hair with the brush. I couldn't tell anyone about this. Brushing was such a natural occurrence. I was embarrassed and ashamed. I was a beautician. I knew the importance of hair care for circulation of the scalp. I got fatigued with simple exertion. Any time I would get spooked, only the left side of my body would jump. When I slept and turned over, I would have to wake up to remember to bring my arm with me. I had to take numerous pills at scheduled times each day. I couldn't stand loud noises, people talking too loud, or loud music. I wanted to isolate myself inside of my home. I would look out the window at the car I used to drive. It was a burgundy 300 ZX. That car was my pride and joy. I would go to my closet just to look at the clothes I used to wear. I would try on different outfits just to try and get a sense of the girl I used to be. Is this going to be what I have to look forward to? No one could possibly know what this feels like to be going through. I felt alone. I was a prisoner locked inside of my own body in this two handed world. Now that the home nurses were cut off by insurance, I was more dependent upon Danny for help. I needed help to take a shower and to use the toilet. I had to get support from him for my waist. My waist had no muscle tone to support my body. He would have to hold my waist and guide me into a sitting position onto the toilet each time I had to go to the bathroom. I had to go frequently. My bladder was severely weakened by the stroke. He had to help me in and out of my wheelchair to sit in the shower chair for my showers. I felt his annoyance growing. It seemed I still couldn't do anything right. To Danny, my paralysis wasn't an excuse. A few weeks went by before I got the strength and the courage to scoot from my wheelchair onto the toilet by myself. After helping me with my shower Danny was in a hurry to go out with his friends for the usual Friday night. I had to use the toilet to relieve my bowels. Danny walked in the bathroom. He yelled, "What are you doing?" I was embarrassed to say. Even in my own home, I had no privacy. Danny was so irate. He started undressing me again. I was still sitting on the toilet. He yelled, "I need to give you another shower because you're dirty again." I felt like his child in training. I found myself in the shower again. I was exhausted from all the scheduled therapy, two showers, and the stress I felt from the man I was engaged to marry. Every night I cried and prayed myself to sleep. I was living a lonely existence. The next morning couldn't have come soon enough. I had a plan to sit outside, in the back yard with my dogs. They were the only things that brought happiness and peace of mind. They loved the fact that they could sit in my lap and go for a ride on my wheelchair. I had to keep up Danny's schedule of therapy exercises. I wheeled myself back into the house. I made up my mind to do any routine or scheduled exercise I was given, I would have a positive attitude about it and complete them. I would read novel after novel to get my eyesight back, and it came back. I would complete 2000 piece puzzles just to get my brain to work. I had to get myself better. I had to get out of there. I wheeled through a puddle on my way inside the house. Our living room had emerald green carpet with white tile that made up the walk ways. This was perfect for my wheel chair. Both tires of my wheelchair made two water lines that stretched the whole length of the white tile, Danny was furious when he woke to see this. His voice rose. He threw a rag at me. "Clean this mess up." I wrapped my right foot around the bottom of my chair to hold on, Inch by inch; I bent over while I sat in my chair. I wiped away the water marks. I was exhausted. I needed a rest, Any exertion after stroke fills your body with exhaustion I wanted to sit on our couch. They were white leather. I wasn't allowed to sit on the couches without a blanket under me; Danny claimed I would dirty his couch. I started at out-patient therapy for occupational therapy. We got the okay from the insurance to go. I needed to find a therapist that cared about me as a person. I was so excited to find someone who could help me get the use of my arm back. My appointment was scheduled for a place called NovaCare Occupational Therapy. Danny wheeled me in the front doors. I was introduced to Jill. She was soft-spoken and middle-aged. She wore glasses that made her look like a school teacher. I felt an immediate connection and peace with her. She explained that she usually worked with pediatrics. My confidence faded. I wasn't a pediatric patient. I was twenty-seven. When am I going to find an occupational therapist that can help my arm? Jill explained to me that when a stroke occurs, the brain develops childlike behavior patterns. These patterns need to be broken. Contractions from spasticity are the main problem. Finally I had found an occupational therapist that could help me, Jill evaluated me and she was confident. She showed me exercises that would strengthen my arm. My therapy lasted for an hour. I took with me a home exercise routine to do daily. She let me borrow her electrical stimulation machine. I would use E-stem after I completed my exercises every day. I saw Jill three times a week: Monday, Wednesday, and Friday. Danny would watch from across the room. Both of his hands were placed on his hips. He wanted to make sure I was working hard enough. I wanted to remember everything Jill said. My short-term memory was a little damaged by the stroke, I wrote down everything. I knew Jill was the one that could help me get some movement from my arm. I had felt this same connection with Bernie. My faith was strong in Bernie since he was the only one to get movement out of my leg. My therapy with Jill finished late one night. Danny and I went out for a late lunch/early dinner at the Denny's across the street. When we arrived home, I was so happy, I found Jill. I sat on the couch, a blanket lay beneath me. I pointed the remote control at the television. I pushed the power button on. A bright light flashed on the television. The television came on, and I passed out. My left side started convulsing first. My whole body followed. I could hear the television. Danny ran in the room. He called 911. I awoke in the Emergency room of the hospital. The neurologist on duty explained that the bright light and flash from the television brought on a seizure. Seizures after a stroke are common. It's a sudden, abnormal electrical activity in the brain. Seizures cause convulsions, tongue biting, falls and frothy sputum. A few minutes passed and I was aware of my surroundings. My energy level was depleted. The medication I was given to counteract the seizures caused an allergic reaction. I itched throughout my whole body. I was sent home with another form of anti-convulsing medication to add to my growing list of medication. Given the new circumstances, I still had the will and the faith to get better. I was looking forward to tomorrow. My friend was going to take me to the mall for some new clothes. I could only buy clothes or shoes I was able to get on by myself. I didn't want to have to need anyone to help me. I was living a lonely existence and I should know how to get dressed alone. I had to pass by the most beautiful clothes at the mall. I could only buy tennis shoes with Velcro. Tennis shoes were the only shoes that would accommodate an orthotic brace. I was a twenty-seven-year-old living as if I were eighty. I was happy with my purchases, I felt like a part of my old self. I knew why I wanted to work so hard to get well. I was given a second chance at life. The paralysis was a setback I had to overcome and win. My friend, Liz, wheeled me in the front door to my home. She said goodbye as she shut the front door. Danny was waiting for me. He said, "I don't want you to live here. I want you to get out. Call your mother. Here's the phone." I was devastated. I was crying so hard I could barely dial the number. I called my mom. She was living with her twin, Lynn. I needed a mother's love at this point. I told her Danny kicked me out and to please come get me. My mom lived twenty minutes away, but only a few minutes had passed when I saw her white Firebird pull to the front of Danny's house. I felt such a relief to see her. I always said she was my best friend but now I knew it, my mother looked just like me with blonde hair. Both Lynn and my mother possessed strength with angelic features, Lynn has always been like a second mother to me. They were happy to see me away from Danny. An intuition told them that there was something not to like about Danny, but couldn't figure out what until now. I felt happy; I could now wake up to the joy of my family's love instead of misery. Strength in the midst of medical problems was something we all shared. Their stories were so extraordinary and similar, it was written in medical journals. My strength was now shadowed by the heaviness of depression. I was grieving for the loss of my left side, for the girl I once was and I now realized Danny's proposal was not meant for true love.

CHAPTER 5

▼

(I can do all things
Through Christ
Which strengtheneth me.)
Philippians 4:13

I woke up with peace of mind in my mom's and aunt's house. I didn't have to struggle to please Danny, from his cleaning, exercising, or controlling manner. I was now to be my sole caregiver, like a mother is to a child. I laid out all of my exercise notes in front of me. I did my first exercise therapy routine for the morning shift. That would only leave noon and evening therapy. This was to be my daily routine. I contacted Bernie and Jill right away. They told me that Danny was continuing payment for their care. This was just another way of looking like the good guy and having me under his thumb. I was seeing both therapists at home five days a week plus doing my own therapy. My days were filled with exercise. The depression weighed so heavily on my shoulders; I missed the girl I once was. How would I support myself in life? My emotions were all over the place. I had to force myself to do each exercise to help my body relearn how to work again. I didn't have a direction; I just knew I had to keep going on. My mom was still heavily into her addition. I was watching this woman I loved and cared for so much become just a shell of her prior self. My paralysis was a huge struggle. My fiancé had left me and I lost the career I loved and had worked so hard to get. I was so emotionally drained, some days I would be fine, then others I would spend my time reading the cards I had saved from the hospital and the journals I wrote in nightly while I was there. I had to read these cards and journals to accept that this stroke really happened to me and to realize my world was falling apart around me. I noticed I wrote three wishes on most of the pages of my journals:

1. Walk again.

2. Get married.

3. Write a book on my stroke.

I was not going to be so gullible again. In the future I wasn't going to let any relationships be based on the realm of disfunction. They would now be centered on honesty. I was going to overcome this stroke and my disabilities. I was realistic in the fact that I knew the brain damage was too great to be as I was. I was going to work hard to get as close to functioning as I could. Now that I was beat down, I had to work my way back up—starting with the wheelchair. It was not what I saw for my future. I was amazed that I was paralyzed, but my back would hurt each time I sat in the chair. Jill told me that my core wasn't strong enough to hold the frame of my body's weight up so my shoulders would slouch and sink into my spine. I started looking in the phone book for disability organizations for housing. I didn't want to have to need anything from anyone. I found a state funded housing called section 8 housing. It was based on how much income you were bringing in. I was getting paid by the state so my income wasn't too much. I located a section 8 housing close to my mom's house, but the list for an apartment was one year long, I put my name on the list. In between therapy, I would be on the phone researching and learning all about state funded organizations for the disabled. I'm the type of person who learns things in detail to get a better understanding of how things work. I worked closely with Jill and Bernie. I felt a real friendship between all of us growing. They couldn't understand why Danny did that to me, except to say that they'd both seen it happen before when significant others, mostly men, were put in the position of caregiver. As much as I wore my brace for my hand continuously, Jill noted that spasticity had set in. I had to fight it, just to get my therapy done. It was exhausting. My spasticity was level 2–3, as written in the Brunnstrom pages for occupational therapy book of terminology. Jill had to give me new exercises as often as the spasticity would increase. The most important thing was, to be aware of the direction of the contractions, and make sure all of my exercises went against it, in the opposite direction. The pain was awful during sleep or therapy. My hand brace had to keep changing along with the exercise plan. With this spasticity I noticed the flacidity starting to be replaced by muscle tone. Jill explained that you don't want spasticity but you have to have a small amount of it to make movement possible after stroke. She said that the brain is like a newborn's brain; the hands want to be in a fist and the arm wants to be bent above the head. It's the brain's way of trying to learn. Without therapy a person could develop bad learning patterns that aren't normal patterns of movement. She said that when I was able to do "angels in the snow" I will have conquered spasticity. I would try and try to do this. I would lie on the mat Jill gave me, and glide my arm upwards in a circular motion. My arm would reach about half way, and then the spasticity would take over my movement, making my arm bend at the elbow towards my face. The spasticity had helped me in the fact that I could move some, but I had too much of it and had to get rid of it. My left side was constantly invaded by pins and needle sensations. Bernie and I worked tirelessly on exercises that would get my core strength stronger, find the middle for equilibrium and weight bearing suitable for walking. Most of our therapy hour revolved around walking out of my wheelchair with my orthotic on, to stabilize my ankle. We walked up and down the block. Bernie was a perfectionist; he would walk closely behind me critiquing every step I made. I would step through with the right foot and then I would step through with the left. I had to make an over-exaggerated circular motion with my hips to put my weight over the left foot. This movement felt exaggerated but looked like a normal step for gait. For weeks, I was only weight bearing on the right foot. I worked and worked on my walking technique. I wanted to be as close to perfect as I could get. Each time I would try to make that switch of weight to the left foot, I would almost fall until Bernie caught me. When a person without a stroke walks, the weight bearing between each foot isn't exaggerated but with a stroke the movements have to be so you can feel the shift of weight happening. Bernie also wanted to teach me how to walk up and down a step. To walk down a step, the stroke side foot had to go first. I had the same feeling in my stomach as when you are at the top of a roller coaster hill, ready to plunge down a hundred foot drop. For the first few tries, I would lose my balance there too, almost falling. Bernie was always there to catch me. To walk up a step, the non-stroke side foot was first. This had to be the way because the strength in my quadriceps and hamstring muscles weren't strong enough to take on my full weight. The day finally came when Bernie was walking behind me, critiquing my steps, and he yelled out, "You have done it!" "Done what?" I asked. "You have taken your first perfect steps." I was so happy. I hugged Bernie, thanking him the whole walk home. My mom folded my wheelchair and put it in the garage. I felt freedom and taller now that I was able to walk out of a wheelchair. I still needed the aide of my orthotic, which was awkward. Every time I would take it off, if I had to go to the bathroom a few feet away, I had to strap it back on. I had to hold my foot in place while grabbing onto the brace with one hand and at the same time strapping it on. If I wanted to relax without the orthotic, I had to think ahead if I had to use the bathroom in the next few minutes. Before my stroke I never had to think if I needed to use the bathroom. I felt I was a cross between an adolescent and an eighty-year-old person. The nights were especially difficult trying to put on the brace when I was half asleep and I had to urinate. Because of the uneven shifts of weight, the brace started rubbing against my skin, breaking it down with each step. After a few short weeks, each step I took was filled with excruciating pain. One day, Bernie and Jill wanted to have a talk with me privately. I thought I was going to hear more bad news because that seemed to be the pattern lately. Bernie was first. He said. "You have got to find the strength to go on with your life alone without Danny. Once they leave, they don't come back." I cried because his words were so harsh. I don't think he got the fact that I was in mourning over the loss of the girl I once was, plus the fabulous career I had to say goodbye to. Jill went next. She told me that with my strength and determination, I had the ability to get much better, but all the stress and worry over my mother and her addiction made her concerned. She had never seen a patient do so well in their recovery and then go in the opposite direction. She asked if I would like to move in with her so we could work harder on therapy. The bond and love I had for my mother was so great, I had to step out of the box of co-dependency so she could find her way to sobriety. With rehab and a lot of hard work, my mother eventually reached sobriety. For the sake of my health, I gladly accepted to move in with Jill. The payments to Bernie and Jill that came from Danny stopped suddenly, I sadly said goodbye to Bernie, the man that changed my life for the better. Bernie had taught me two things—one was to walk, and the other was not to judge a book by its cover. As a surprise, my mother bought me a ticket to go see my step-sister, June, in Lake Tahoe. My mother has always been there for me. As strong as her addiction was, she had saved her money for a plane ticket for me. It broke her heart to see the sadness in me and thought a trip to Lake Tahoe would do me good. I wasn't looking forward to this trip, some days I felt too depressed to move. The next weekend I moved in with Jill. She picked me up. I was excited to get working hard on my therapy. Jill was married with four kids, a boy and three girls. I would sleep in her middle daughter Morgan's room for the duration of my stay. We pulled up in Jill's mini van; her family gave me a warm greeting. They were used to their mother's patients. A few years before, Jill helped a girl who had a traumatic brain injury after a car accident. She made a full recovery with Jill's help. Jill and I started with therapy right away. She taught me how to fold clothes and stir food contents in a bowl with one hand; I had to use a plastic mat called a dycem sheet to prevent the bowl from moving with each stir. She taught me how to use a one handed can opener and jar opener, and how to chop food. The cutting board had two nails sticking out of the top to stabilize the food item while cutting. The knife was called a rocker knife that had a rounded edge to rock back and forth. My routine for the day would be my own therapy in the morning, two walks up and down the block, and in the afternoon I would work on household duties like vacuuming, laundry, folding and making small meals to learn kitchen habits. I noticed the times when I was alone I would feel panicked and a loss of breath, every tingle or pin feeling in my left arm would send a terror through me. The night that I had the seizure at Danny's house, Danny was out of the room. My left hand had a tingling sensation when the seizure hit my nervous system. I was terrified to have another one because I could hear and see what was going on, but didn't have any control over my body and I could not speak. It felt like I was trapped under water and couldn't get out. After Jill would get home from work, she and I would work on occupational therapy plus pool therapy. Jill later told me her kids loved living with me but got jealous of all of the attention she gave me. Jill was much more than a therapist to me; she was a friend, a mentor, the one who brought God's presence back into my life and the one who taught me how to love myself again. Christmas came while living with Jill. She gave me a white robe (just like my favorite movie star Marilyn Monroe wore in one of her movies) and a letter which read as follows ...

12/19/95 Dear Renee,
How do I begin saying adequately just how much I have enjoyed getting to know you this past year. You are such a lovely, wonderful person and some day, hopefully soon, you will realize that in many ways the disabilities you are now facing have helped bring you out of your finite, sheltered, and comfortable world into a blend with humanity you would have never known. Life is dependent on how we make it. It is not dependent on how we look or how we move. It's on how we react to one another. Lives are like whispers in time. We are here then we are gone, the choices we make are what drives our eternity. You've made a difference in my life. I am better for having known you,
Love always in Christ,
Jill

I ate dinner at my mom's and aunt's house each weekend. We discussed my upcoming trip to Lake Tahoe. I told them how much I didn't want to go because I was just too depressed to see myself doing anything fun. My aunt said, "If you don't get on that plane, I will never talk to you again. I want you to get a break and to see you have fun again." I received a letter in the mail from the section 8 housing apartments, Sunrise Manner. I could move in any time. I would share a common living area and kitchen with three elderly men. My rent was $150.00 a month, utilities $30.00, and the phone was $15.00. I had called Danny to ask for all of my belongings back, my dogs, and if he could sell my car, so I could have some money to buy furniture. He said he wasn't giving me back my dogs because he bought them, but he could get my car sold. My car sold in a couple weeks. Danny gave my $2500.00 to Gina (now his sister-in-law) to give to me. Jill drove me around to purchase furniture for my one-bedroom apartment. I bought a white lacquer full size bedroom set, a 19 inch television set, a two person table, and a VCR. Jill helped me with the move into Sunrise Manner the next weekend. We hugged each other and said goodbye. She told me what she thought of me. She thought I was courageous, and a very special human being, a gentle, sweet, loving, and kind person. We knew that we would always have a friend in each other. My friend, Liz, helped me pick up my things from Danny's house. Danny already had his new girlfriend Tara living there. No one was home when Liz and I got there, not even my dogs. We walked into the house and my belongings were scattered everywhere in the living room. At my apartment, I made friends with all of the elderly people living there; they all called me their granddaughter. The complex offered lunch; I would eat my lunches with all of the elderly and played bingo afterwards each day together. 1/8/96, my mom dropped me off at McCarran airport for my flight to Reno. My step-sister June picked me up. June was my step-dad's second daughter from a previous marriage, I felt close to June. She was so excited to see me; I used to see her every summer, when I was a kid. We drove the hour to Lake Tahoe. The drive was so beautiful. Peace came over me as we drove over the hill and I saw serene Lake Tahoe. The Lake was huge and turquoise blue in color. June explained to me that she was renting a room from her boss, Kevin. We pulled up to the two story, green, ranch style house. June told me her bedroom was a separate apartment upstairs, but she wanted to introduce me to her boss first. In my orthotic, I was able to climb the three stairs before the front door. I walked in and I noticed Kevin sitting at the table. He was wearing Levis, a sweatshirt, and a baseball cap. The paper was opened up to the sports section. June had told me he was the poker manager at Harvey's casino where she worked. June introduced us, and we shook hands. His eyes met mine, his welcome was warm. Kevin recognized me from my modeling pictures June showed him prior to my arrival. While looking at my pictures, all he could think of was that this girl was a beautiful, Las Vegas girl, who would never be interested in him. He felt an immediate connection with me now though. Before him wasn't the snobbish, Las Vegas girl, he had imagined. I felt my heart flutter just to look at him and oddly, I felt an immediate crush on this man I just met. Kevin later told me he felt the same exact way. I thought to myself after all the bad relationships I've had, I don't want to like this man and how could I already have a crush on him?

I asked Kevin for some aspirin to relieve the headache I had from the drive up. The doctors told me I would always have bad headaches due to the massive brain swelling. Kevin handed me the aspirin, and then I turned around and walked with June upstairs. Kevin watched me walk the distance across the living room to June's door. I told June I'd like to get to know that man better, and I was hoping that if he saw that I had to wear braces on my hand and foot he wouldn't be turned off by it. I wore my brace in the day hours to keep the spasticity from contracting into painful positions. June said he didn't want to date anyone because he was going through a terrible divorce. After he and his wife had three children, they lost interest in each other. After she had the kids, she tried controlling his every move from limiting his golf outings with the guys to forbidding him to enjoy a drink after work among other things. She told him if he stayed out after work one more time, she would leave. He saw a way out of the marriage and stayed out until the early hours of the morning. When he got home, she had taken the kids and all household items; he was left with nothing except some utensils for cooking. He received divorce papers from an attorney a week later. I didn't sleep the whole night because I was thinking of Kevin. I thought of different scenarios of how I could get to know him better. June had told me what time he left for work, 9:00am. I woke up early; I was hoping I would casually run into him to start a conversation. I opened June's door, and I was stunned. Kevin was sitting just a few feet in front of me on the couch. The television was showing a baseball game and he was reading the sports section. I knew nothing about sports except that my dogs and I weren't allowed in the room when Danny watched them because we were bad luck. I asked who he was rooting for.

He said, "It doesn't matter." Our conversation flowed; I never had a problem talking with people.

The night before my return home, I woke up early to write Kevin a note to tell him how beautiful his house was, how much I liked his dog, Mia, and to thank him for his hospitality of letting me stay in his home. June directed me to his room; I would leave my note on his pillow. I walked in his room. The room was a mess from front to back. I thought he would never see my note in all the disarray. I knew the best way to a man's heart was through his stomach, but that wasn't one of my strengths. My strength was neatness. I would have to rely on that. I made the bed, vacuumed the room, dusted the tables, put the clothes back in their drawers, wiped down the mirrors, scrubbed the toilet and sink, and then I left my note on his pillow, along with my number. My note read as follows …

Kevin,

A letter of thanks to you. The stay at your home has been a pleasant delight. Your house is beautiful and the feelings of happiness when I'm here I can't describe.

Thank you for your warm hospitality. I'm glad I got the chance to meet you.

Renee

P.S. If you don't want your dog,
Here's my number #220–3301

June drove me to the airport the next morning. The whole flight I was thinking I didn't want to like this man and get hurt when he didn't call. My heart pounded each time I thought of him but I had to protect my heart. My mom was waiting for me at the airport to drive me to my apartment. I got ready for bed and tried my hardest not to think of Kevin. I wrote in my journal … Kevin from Lake Tahoe is nice but I don't like him. My phone rang at 8:00pm. Kevin was on the other end of the line; he wanted to thank me for cleaning his room. I was so shocked that he called and so elated to be talking to him again. We talked for four hours; he invited me to come back to Lake Tahoe on Valentine's Day, the next month. I ecstatically accepted. We talked every night three to four hours. I never tired of hearing his voice. I didn't trust Kevin until each time he would say he would call, he did. Each time he said he would do something, he did. He was honest and a man of his word. I received the plane ticket from Kevin in the mail; our first date would be Valentine's Day. I heard of a state funded organization for brain injured persons called Nevada Community Enrichment Program (NCEP). This organization was designed to teach brain injured persons to get back into the world. They taught cooking skills, therapy exercises, vocational needs, and psychology therapy. My application papers were denied because I was not disabled enough. I was disappointed but this was another fight I had to overcome, after all I was disabled, I needed all the help I could get to get my life back. I needed a brace to walk, my arm still hung by my side, I had partial movement in my bicep, and no movement from my fingers. I called the manager of NCEP every day to see if he would change his mind. I wasn't going to let them take away any opportunities I might have at getting my life back. The answer was NO for a month, until the manager of NCEP didn't want to keep hearing from me every day, he said I was enrolled. I would have to get there at 8:00am, without being late. My name was written on a board in the main room. I would have a different class every hour, but my interest was mainly in the occupational therapy they offered. All I thought about was getting my arm stronger and getting back to the job I loved. I would leave NCEP at 4:30pm every day. I contacted a friend, Dan, at the salon where I used to work. I asked if he needed an assistant to clean up after each job or sweep hair. If I had to start at the bottom, I would. Dan said I could start work right away. Since I didn't drive, I had to take the bus for the disabled, Paratransit, to get to NCEP and then to my job with Dan. After I left NCEP at 4:30pm, I would get a ride over to work with Dan from 5pm to 8pm. Dan paid me by the job. In between sweeping I would stare at my empty station. I had to hold my tears back from forming. I went home each night exhausted. I would have to take my bath before bed each night because I had to be at NCEP by 8:00am. I had to sit in a chair next to the bathtub, take my brace off, scoot from the chair to the edge of the bathtub, then scoot down slowly into the water by holding onto the edge of the tub with one hand.

To get out, I had to lift my body with my right hand. Once I was at the edge of the tub, I scooted back onto the chair so I could dry off and put my brace on. Getting dressed with one hand took a long time so I had to get dressed before I went to bed. Taking a bath wasn't the enjoyable experience it used to be and now sleeping wasn't comfortable either, dressed in clothes for the next day. I cried every night and prayed the same prayer. "God, please help make me a wife, please find my husband for me." I could only keep up the schedule of going to NCEP and working for Dan for two months. I was exhausted. My life had completely changed, I still mourned for the girl I once was but I felt a certain sense of peace to be away from Danny.

2/14/96, I left for Reno. June picked me up because Kevin had to work. We drove to Lake Tahoe and I met Kevin at Harvey's. He had a red rose and an angel book waiting on his desk as a gift. He knew I loved angels. I walked in and we hugged and kissed each other. The month we waited to see each other seemed like an eternity. I felt safe and peaceful in his arms; I never wanted to be away from him again. I thought this was the kindest, gentlest soul I had ever known. June was a poker dealer and worked under Kevin. She said she and everyone working under him felt the same way.

Kevin made reservations to have dinner at the gourmet room at Harvey's casino, The Sage Room. Kevin warned me that because it was Lake Tahoe, people would ask if I had been in a ski accident. Kevin had a ski accident in 1980. He went off a jump, landed wrong, and flipped backwards on his head. The ski patrol said he was comatose for forty-five minutes but released him to go home. Later that night, he went to dinner with a friend, Michelle. She could tell something was terribly wrong with Kevin's brain in his speech patterns and thought process. Michelle rushed Kevin to the emergency room at Barton Memorial Hospital. The neurologist gave him CAT scans to determine what had happened in his brain. In the accident, his brain was shaken like Jell-O, he had a concussion, his neck was sprained, and he was convulsing with seizures. The doctors didn't know what his chances were for life; he was admitted into Intensive Care.

The waitress came to take our order and the first thing she asked was if I had a ski accident. Kevin and I laughed; I reluctantly explained what had happened to me. I didn't want for the stroke to be a replacement for me. I was a person outside of the stroke. A professional photographer came over after the waitress left to take our first picture together. The dinner was delicious; I had a pasta dish because I didn't want to ask for Kevin's help to cut anything. Kevin had filet mignon. We talked and laughed through the whole meal, continuing our romantic flirting back and forth all the way home that night. Kevin was only ten years my senior and not like any other man I had ever met. I knew we were falling in love. I flew back and forth to see Kevin two more times. In between these visits, we were on the phone to each other. Each conversation we would talk for three or four hours about nothing. In one conversation, Kevin told me he loved me. I answered back by telling him I couldn't say the same yet because of every thing I had been through in my past, he told me he understood. On the last visit to see Kevin, we sat on the couch in front of the fireplace, the moon shining through the huge windows of the living room. Our relationship felt comfortable, safe, and every other sentence brought out laughter in both of us. Kevin told me how much he loved me. I knew I wasn't going to just date someone for years without a commitment so I told him that, and I told him of my wishes to be married. Kevin asked me to marry him. I said no because I felt I was forcing the issue by telling him my wishes.

The next morning I flew back to Las Vegas. My every thought was on Kevin and the question of marriage. I needed my mom's advice at this point. I went for dinner at her house and asked, "Do you think it would be safe for me to love this man and say yes?" My mother and aunt recognized a happiness they hadn't seen in years. They both said yes and it was okay to let down my guard and say yes to marriage. I ate my dinner so fast, I didn't even remember chewing my food. I told my mom I wanted to hurry and go home to call Kevin. I called Kevin and said, "Remember when I told you no, to your marriage Proposal? Well … can I change my answer to a yes?" Kevin sounded so happy through the phone. I could almost hear him smiling. Kevin said yes. We were engaged. God answered my prayers.

CHAPTER 6

▼

(What has happened to me will turn out for
My deliverance)
Philippians 1:19

I continued my routine of catching the Paratransit (bus for the disabled) for a ride to NCEP. I started outgrowing this facility of therapy. Most of the patients were so badly brain damaged. One boy shot himself through his frontal lobe after his girlfriend broke up with him, but didn't die. He would walk around in a daze crying when he should have laughed or laughing when he heard something sad. Another man was in a fight and was jumped by two other men. He fell and hit the back part his head damaging the brain. He walked around in complete confusion of who he was or where he was. There were car accident brain injuries and one other elderly stroke survivor. NCEP kept coupling my brain injury together with the more serious cases of brain injury. I had always been very organized and a multi-tasked person yet NCEP counselors told me this was my brain injury affecting me because I couldn't concentrate on one task at a time. I always felt I needed to make my bed before leaving in the morning. The counselors told me this was my brain injury affecting me because I didn't have the ability to let something go for a day. I was feeling aggravated because I held all of these same characteristics prior to my stroke and brain injury. Again, I grew concerned over the treatment for my arm. The occupational therapist would treat the more severe brain injured patients just because it was their assigned job to treat any patient who sat in front of them. My problems were mostly motor skills. I felt my arm needed more attention than just the twenty minutes the therapist would spare in between patients. After NCEP, each day I would go home, lay out my old notes from Jill and do my own occupational therapy. I would do my exercises until I would get too physically tired to do anymore. NCEP was putting together a talent show for the patients. The counselors wanted to see me involved with doing hair again. My part in the show was to make over one of the counselors. I had two goals to reach at NCEP. The first goal was to win this talent show and receive the award. After a lot of thought and effort in doing this project with one hand, I won the contest. My other goal was to complete my stay at NCEP, graduate and receive my certificate of completion. Once a month I had to meet with counselors to talk over my progress but they were concerned when I told them I met someone. They didn't want me falling in the same pattern of getting hurt by someone. I felt obligated to agree with everything they said because if I didn't, they would blame my brain injury on not thinking the way I should and prolong my stay. NCEP taught me how to be self-assured about living in the world with paralysis. They taught cooking skills, how to use my quadriceps as another arm to help hold objects so I could open them, and how to love the person I was. Once a month I had to get CAT scans on my brain. They checked to see if there were any changes. Stroke survivors are at a high risk of suffering another stroke for up to five years after the first one. The average is twenty-four percent of recurring stroke for women and forty-two percent for men. I felt I was just going through the motions of pretending to be happy after stroke and paralysis, because the depression and grieving over the girl I once was never left me. It felt as though my heart was crying silent tears but my lips would be smiling so others wouldn't be able to tell how I really felt. The NCEP counselors told me severe depression after stroke is very common in the first stages of recovery and years following. My depression got so severe some nights; unsure thoughts of whether or not to stay on this earth ran across my mind frequently. I hated feeling like that because I knew in my heart how much I loved life. I knew I had to turn to my faith for guidance. I was invited to go to church by a girl I worked with at the salon. We would go every Wednesday night, and that's where I met Pastor Reggie. He preached on a non-denominational faith, it felt like every sermon he would preach, he was talking to me. After each sermon, I made a point of staying to talk with Pastor Reggie to get his insight on these terrible feelings I was invaded with. Pastor Reggie reassured me that my life had a purpose and meaning. He told me that God was with me in every aspect of my life and was working behind the scenes for a better future.

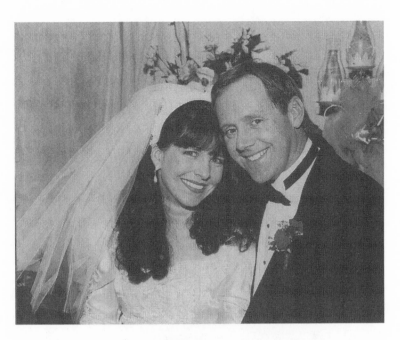

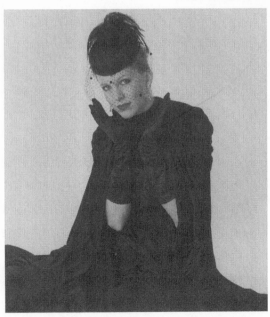

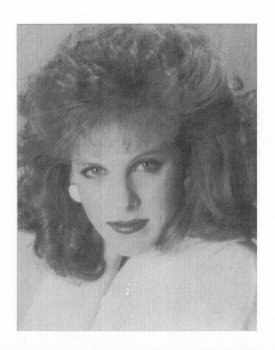

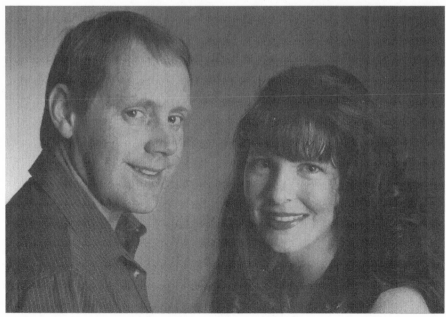

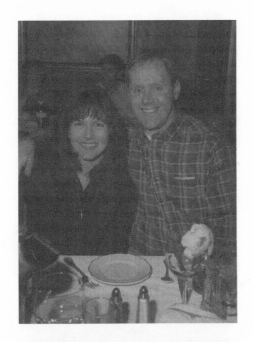

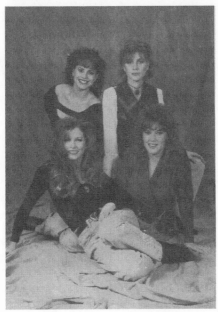

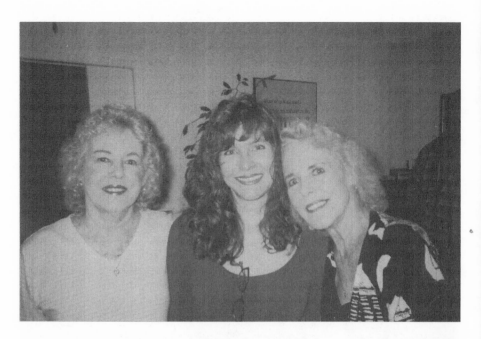

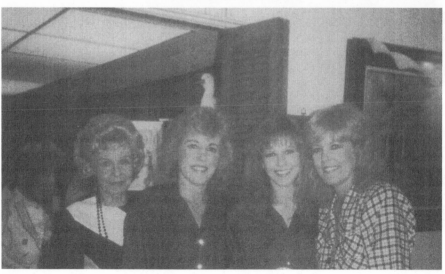

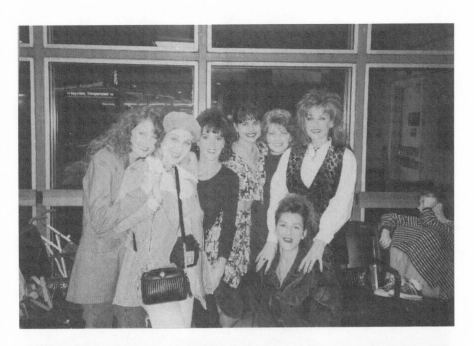

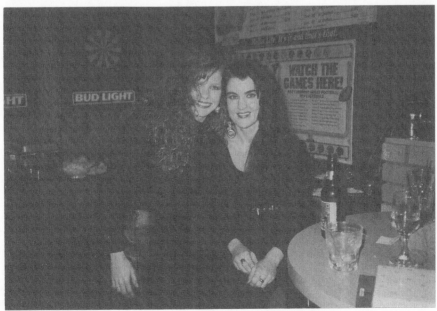

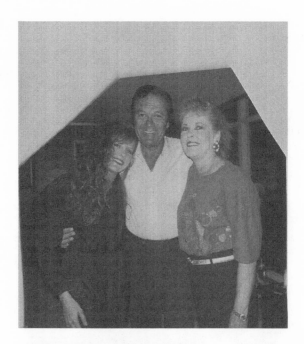

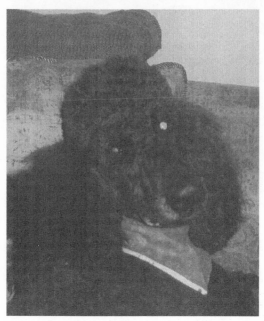

There was always a bright light that would shine on all of the grief and depression I felt constantly, and that was Kevin. He and I carried on our long distance relationship, getting to know each other more in depth for months. Kevin never missed a night of calling me. The love that we had between us grew, and we longed for the day when we could be together again. One phone call, I could sense the frustration in Kevin's voice. He told me he had enough of the distance that separated us. He was going to drive up and bring me back with him to Lake Tahoe to live. I was looking forward to Kevin's arrival, but I had to complete my goal of receiving my certificate of completion for graduation from NCEP. Kevin's plan was to drive all night, after working on Thursday from Lake Tahoe to Las Vegas. We would attend my graduation, pack up the U-Haul he rented, and we would drive back to Lake Tahoe together. I graduated from NCEP and received my certificate. I learned that my brain injury didn't take away from the person I was, and this was God's way of closing a door so he could open a window. When we arrived in Lake Tahoe, the snow was falling. It continued falling the whole night and the whole weekend. I was not used to this kind of weather raised in Las Vegas. Kevin and I walked outside to a snow that was taller than me, I'm five foot six. Through the weeks I noticed that spasticity started settling into my leg and foot. My steps would be robotic like and rigid, along with my foot dropping in a downwards position making walking extremely painful. I had drop foot. Drop foot is paralysis or weakness of the dorsiflexor muscles of the foot and ankle resulting in dragging of the foot and toes.

(1996)—Achilles tendon lengthening surgery—My mom researched and found a doctor in Las Vegas that does this procedure. About a month after I moved to Lake Tahoe, I flew back to Las Vegas for tendon lengthening day surgery. About seventy-five percent of the patients will be able to walk out of the orthotic brace. Recurrence of the foot deformity will occur in fifteen percent of stroke patients. While my foot healed up from surgery, I could not weight bear on my foot for a week. The pain was extreme the first and second day after surgery but decreased in the days following. I couldn't wait to get back to Kevin and try walking without the painful orthotic brace I'd worn for months. After the surgery healed I was only able to walk without the orthotic some of the time for short distance walking. I still needed the aide of the orthotic to stabilize my ankle for walking. I went to physical therapy thirty minutes away in Carson City twice a week because the insurance from the state only approved therapy facilities in Carson City for that area. I did my own occupational therapy three times a week for my arm.

I had to start planning my wedding. Kevin worked all the time so all the plans and correspondence was left up to me. Organization of the wedding details and plans was a full time job, but trying to fit everything into a day was hard. Doing my exercises for my leg, then different exercises for my arm, walking, calling the wedding hall, making payments to the wedding hall, getting Kevin's family's addresses from all across the state of Nevada, and being the wife I knew I could be to Kevin was my daily routine. Kevin's idea was to have our wedding on the same date as my stroke three years later 5/3/97. He wanted to make this day better for me. I got a call from my Aunt Lynn, telling me doctors had just found a large mass in my mother's stomach, and she was being scheduled for surgery because of how serious her condition was. After a full hysterectomy, doctors diagnosed her tumor as stage four, the worst stage with cancer you could have. She would need chemotherapy and weekly blood transfusions. I was devastated and feared for my mother's life. Under the worst of circumstances, my mother routinely sent monetary gifts to provide Kevin and me with the finances for a beautiful wedding. After four blood transfusions, my mother was able to attend our wedding. My friend Gina called me in Lake Tahoe to tell me my dog (now Danny's dog) Ginger was having puppies. I felt I deserved a dog from Ginger. I called Danny and practically begged for a puppy from Ginger's litter. Kevin and I drove down to see the dogs, and Danny reluctantly handed over a tiny apricot poodle. I named her Mocha. Kevin and I had to drive down periodically to take marriage classes from Pastor Reggie. I was going to do everything I could to make my marriage last. On one trip to Las Vegas, we left Mocha with a friend of Kevin's. When we arrived back home he let us know he thought Mocha had died. He said she got outside during a bad snow storm, and the only thing he could see was a bunch of coyotes around the area. We all presumed a coyote got Mocha. I cried day and night for Mocha and my mother. I searched for Mocha every chance I could until I had to accept she was gone. I had to pull myself together because I still had wedding details to finish and it was important to me to be a supportive wife to Kevin. I had a bridal shower in Lake Tahoe with Kevin's family a couple weeks before our planned trip to Las Vegas and another in Las Vegas with my family. The week before the wedding Kevin and I flew to Las Vegas. Our services were going to be held in a wedding hall that provided all the services: the ceremony, flowers, video, pictures, reception hall, food, and a three tiered cake. My only request was to have Pastor Reggie marry us; he was the one who brought the joy of life back into my life. I had to walk down the isle to the man I loved wearing an orthotic brace and tennis shoes that my wedding dress covered. I was thrilled to be marrying a man that truly loved me, paralysis or not.

CHAPTER 7

▼

(Choosing to be positive is
going to determine how
you're going to live your life.)
Joel Osteen

Kevin and I honeymooned in Mexico. This was the wedding gift from Kevin's parents to us. It was an expense paid stay at their time share at the Pueblo Bonito Resort Hotel. Our room overlooked tropical grounds, a pool, and the breathtaking ocean. On the grounds, the first thing that caught my eye as an extreme animal lover was the flamingos walking around, and an iguana that rested near our patio. I was living a happiness I never knew existed. We wanted to go outside to enjoy the beautiful grounds of The Pueblo Bonito, especially the bar inside of the pool. We hurriedly got dressed in our bathing suits. I was excited because this was the first new bathing suit I had purchased in three years since having a stroke. Before my suit was completely on, Kevin commented on how beautiful I looked. I felt beautiful and smiled as I walked to the mirror. I looked at myself in the bathing suit and my heart dropped. Once again I felt my silent tears streaming. The suit looked beautiful but I knew I would be the only girl walking around the grounds wearing an orthotic and tennis shoes. I had to swallow my sadness because I also knew I would be walking hand in hand with the most wonderful man in Mexico.

Once at the pool, I had to unstrap the orthotic and leave it and my tennis shoes by the side of the pool while we got in. I felt relief when I didn't need Kevin's help to stay afloat, the weightlessness of the water made it possible for me to walk normally. I thought, at least I could be able-bodied for a short period while walking in water.

After a time in the pool, we went for a short walk down by the ocean. I was looking forward to showing Kevin a popular tourist bar called Senior Frogs to top our day off that evening. We ate dinner at the hotel restaurant and headed for Senior Frogs bar. When we walked in, the whole place was crawling with wall to wall tourists; the music was playing loudly with tourists dancing on the dance floor. We sat in a booth, I ordered my signature one beer and Kevin had his drink. Like the day by the pool, I was wearing my orthotic and tennis shoes. I had to ignore the stares I was getting while Kevin and I got up to dance. I needed help from Kevin to stand up while I tried to move my hips to look like dancing. I didn't want my disability to get in the way of Kevin's good time. My balance wasn't good when it came to something my brain wasn't used to such as dancing.

After ten minutes of pretending to dance, I had to sit down while Kevin went to the bathroom. I headed for a bench to rest and my unsteady balance got the best of me. Before I reached the bench, my legs gave way and I fell to the floor. As much as I had fallen before, I still couldn't get used to the piercing pain that passed through my body when my body hit the hard surface each time. No one bothered to help me up, they probably thought I had one to many. With my one hand, I managed to pull myself onto a bench nearby. When Kevin came out of the bathroom, I told him what had happened. He felt terrible that he was gone at that moment. I felt like a clam who wanted to withdraw into its shell, but I wasn't going to let that unfortunate occurrence steal my joy from being in love with my husband and the time we were having together. We stayed a little while longer listening to music and got our picture taken from a photographer for a memory to have from Senior Frogs. Our stay in Mexico was so romantic, but on the seventh day we had to check out of room #214 at the Pueblo Bonito to go back to reality, and start our new lives together. The love I felt for Kevin filled my whole body with joy and happiness. My stroke took my movement but God brought the love of Kevin into my life. Once back in Lake Tahoe, I got back to my routine of doing my own therapy and once a week driving down to Carson City for outpatient therapy. I thought it was time for me to look for a job. I applied to any job I thought I could do with one hand—receptionist, and administrative assistant—getting rejected from every interview. I tried applying for a hostess job at the casino restaurant at the casino where Kevin worked, keeping in mind that I didn't have experience in this field. I wanted to contribute as much to the marriage as I could. Kevin knew the manager at the restaurant and had an interview set up. The interview went extremely well with the manager and me. When Kevin came home later from work, he gave me the news. The manager of the restaurant told him he liked me, and my personality would be perfect for hostessing but he just didn't feel that with one hand that I could handle the job. I would have to stay home to continue therapy on my own. The instincts of motherhood were starting to invade my thoughts more frequently. Kevin and I made an appointment to see an OBGYN. We had a few things that were against us conceiving a child. Kevin had a vasectomy after having three children from his previous marriage, of whom he saw three times a month; his heart wasn't into having another child. The doctor told me at no time should I ever have children. I would have another stroke or die trying to give birth. On the drive home, I was disappointed but somehow knew that this wasn't the best path to take for our marriage. I wanted to follow every dream of having a child as every woman does but my true love was what was best for my husband. I did long for the love and care of an animal though. I read that caring for an animal after surviving a stroke can increase your chances of getting well faster, and that an animal's love had the ability to decrease depression.

I was on two different types of seizure medication at this time and seizure free for months. One night Kevin and I had dinner at the casino where he worked and then we decided to take a walk through the casino so he could introduce me to his friends. I felt my left arm and fingers moving, which was a warning sign for a seizure in my body. I turned to warn Kevin and just as soon as I got the words out, "I'm going to have a seizure," my body was filled with terror, claustrophobia, and a panicked feeling of not being able to breathe, and then the convulsions violently started. I could hear Kevin yell out to a security guard, "Go get Carlos the doctor out of the poker room." Carlos stopped his poker playing and ran up to me, put his jacket under my head and comforted me until the paramedics arrived. I was rushed to Barton Memorial Hospital emergency room. The neurologist assessed my situation by giving me a CAT scan. The results came back as seizure disorder brought on by stress and the slot machine bells in the casino. I was now prescribed a third medication just to control the breakthrough seizures because of my massive brain injury after my stroke. I felt like my stroke and my disability were trying to stop me from fulfilling some of the dreams every girl has. Kevin received a call from a friend who knew of a friend opening up a new card room in the bay area. They needed a top man to run this poker room and Kevin was his first thought.

The room needed employees of all sorts and the money he would bring in would be better than what he was receiving presently. Kevin asked if there was a job I could possibly do. There was a PBX operator/administrative assistant opening that would be suitable for me because this could be done with one hand. Kevin and I were planning a move to the bay area. Kevin and I drove to and from the bay area in hopes of finding a place to rent. On one trip down Kevin surprised me with a detour to Napa Valley. He told me to look for a dog breeder for standard poodles because he knew I loved the standard poodle breed. Kevin and I drove to a small groomers shop and all you could see were standard poodles—adult poodles of every color and a litter of black balls of fur standard poodles. My heart was filled with joy to feel the love of an animal again. One little girl puppy was attached to me; we took her home and I named her Holly for holly-berries at Christmas season since Christmas was around the corner. Kevin went to the bay area ahead of me to start work while I packed the house up. A month later I joined him. Once in the bay area, I started working as a PBX operator. I was so elated to be working again; I helped out in any department of the card room that needed it. My favorite was human resources because that had the most interaction with the employees. I worked the swing shift and thrived. I soon learned the names, employees, and departments of all three hundred employees. My parents always taught me it was good to have a career to fall back on so during the day, I enrolled in the local community college to try and get an education in a field I could do with one hand. I took classes three times a week to complete an associate degree, and worked five nights a week swing shift at the card room. I raced home each day just to see Holly. She was the child I couldn't have. This was getting to be a regular with my life, the dreams I had were taken away from me by the stroke but being replaced by alternate things. I walked so much on the grounds of the college and at work that the orthotic started rubbing again with every unbalanced sway of my gait. The skin around my ankle started breaking down into huge sores. Every step I took, severe pain would race through my body. I made an appointment after school one day to see a podiatrist. I didn't have high hopes of this doctor helping me because I already had the ankle tendon lengthening surgery and it didn't work. Dr. Dobbs walked in and he was young and friendly. I was polite but had little faith in what he could do for my situation. He asked a question everyone seemed to ask me, why I had a stroke so young. He looked at my foot, and then excused himself from the room. Twenty minutes later, I thought this doctor forgot me, until he walked back in the room. He asked if I thought about surgery. I said, "Can you make me walk without the orthotic?" Dr. Dobbs replied. "Do you want minor or major surgery?" I said, "Anything that could help me walk without the aide of the orthotic."

Dr. Dobbs said, "This would be major surgery."

2000—Ankle fusion/tendon lengthening—Fusing the foot and ankle bones into a functional position to relieve pain and to omit the orthotic. Recovery would mean no weight bearing for a period of six weeks. A month before the surgery, Dr. Dobbs had me be the guest at the foot clinic he taught at so he could teach future podiatrists what happens to the foot and gait after stroke. After the surgery I awoke in the recovery room and a violent wave of pain pounded through my nervous system. I cried out in pain. I spent the next three nights in the hospital. Any inch of movement I would make would start a chain reaction of pain through my body. My mother came to my side as I was released from the hospital. I found myself sitting back in a wheelchair. Because of the pain, it was impossible for me to bathe, brush my teeth or do anything that was functioning. I needed the help from my mother. I was like a child all over again. I didn't want to take a chance of putting any weight through my ankle. I had to have this surgery work. Having this surgery meant I had to give up school because of the help I would need and the wheelchair I would be in for six weeks. I went to school to talk with my counselor a couple weeks before the surgery to remove my name from my classes. My counselor was concerned and sat me down to explain how much she didn't think I should quit because in all of my classes I was making A's & B's. I explained how important this surgery was to me; I had to withdraw my name, and walked out of school.

I was starting to get used to the depression every time I had to give up things or dreams I had. Six weeks passed and I had to start six weeks of therapy for my foot and to now get used to my foot and walking with my foot in a functional position minus constant pain. As usual I incorporated my own therapy while at home. After my foot healed from the surgery, I was finally able to wear other styles of shoes besides tennis shoes; I was starting to feel more like myself. My ankle would never have the strength to hold my weight in a high heal shoe. I tried but my ankle failed causing a painful fall to the ground each time I tried. We had been working at the casino for three years 98–00, when we realized that the bay area's cost of living was too much for us to afford. Kevin and I planned the move back to Nevada where we could get back on our feet. We couldn't move back to Lake Tahoe because of the lack of job opportunities for me so we decided on Reno, Nevada. Word of mouth found Kevin looking for a job in the Reno/Lake Tahoe area and he was hired right away in the poker room of his former employer. It took me six months when I was hired at a local department store's cosmetic counter. I informed the store manager of my background. I was hired right away. I made sure I clearly explained to the manager of the cosmetic counter about my disability and that I would need periodic sitting breaks. There was a lot more to this job than just selling products. I stocked, lifted heavy boxes, organized shelves, and sold and returned clothing from the department area. I got fatigued quicker than usual at this job because of all of the standing and lifting. I started making small errors in the returns of products or clothing. I wanted to do the best I could and asked the manager if I could go back through training on the register just to know the area of returning better. I won an award for great customer service skills. I worked at this job seven months when I was called into the manager's office. We talked about the area of returns and she pointed to her head with two of her fingers and said because of what happened to me with my stroke, I was unable to do this job. "We are terminating you as of today." I was so hurt because of the fact I let her know when I was hired I was disabled, and I tried to overcome the problem I had by going back through register training. I contacted Equal Rights for the disabled. I filled out exactly what had happened and I was told there would be a phone meeting with an arbitrator as the go between for Equal Rights. I was nervous but kept my cool and told the truth. The conversation got very quiet when I explained the part about how the manager held up her two fingers, pointed to her head, and said because of what happened to me, I couldn't do the job. I won the argument and felt proud to be fighting for my rights.

I was still walking without the aide of the orthotic and extremely happy because of this. I wrote Dr. Dobbs a thank you letter every year on the anniversary of the ankle fusion surgery. I wanted Dr. Dobbs to know how thankful I was and how he had changed my life for the better. Dr. Dobb's surprisingly wrote me back on an occasion saying ...

With every letter you write me I feel so honored to have been a part in helping you move on with your life. Your thoughts are an inspiration to me and are in no small part the reason surgeons do what they do. Helping you has been perhaps my most rewarding accomplishments in over 30—years of surgery.
Fondly,
Dr. Dobbs

I applied for Medicare/social security getting turned down again. I supported myself through unemployment. This went on for a year when I landed a job at a real-estate company as their receptionist. Once again, I explained thoroughly that I was disabled, and after the second interview I was hired. I loved working around people. I answered the phones, made packets, did spread sheets on the computer and volunteered for any other work the agents might need. Once a week different agents would sit in a booth behind my desk to answer the incoming calls from buyers. One male agent, Adam, would demand to have things done from me quickly and for the calls to be put through quicker. It finally got to the point of insulting. I complained to the boss of the company and there was a meeting between us three. I asked if Adam was my boss and if I had to listen to him. I was told I only had to assist him in areas of need but that I didn't have to listen to him as if he were my boss. Matters between Adam and I did not change, in fact got worse and escalated to a point of irate anger at me because I wasn't moving fast enough for him. I complained again to the boss with no change from Adam. After three years on that job I was terminated because the corporation behind the company thought Adam was a money maker because he was a realtor and should be kept over me. Again I contacted Equal Rights. A meeting was set up in person this time with an arbitrator. I was so nervous but I felt I was fighting for the rights for the disabled, as a disabled woman. I told the truth. The arbitrator told me he couldn't believe the reasons behind Adam and his anger because I dressed well, spoke well, and was a very professional and articulate woman. I won my case through the help of Equal Rights for the disabled. I applied to Medicare/social security again because I needed some help from the government to support myself. I was turned down again. A poem I wrote ...

<u>Yesterday I cried</u>
Yesterday I cried
I thought about the
Person I once was,
I told myself I didn't miss her,
I lied.
When I woke, numbness replaced my left side,
What's wrong with me?
Hemorrhagic stroke, I can't feel,
Independence I no longer have.
Is this a nightmare?
No ... It's real.
Acceptance I have tried,
I said goodbye to you,
A new me has risen,
Yesterday I cried.

I had to be diligent about all of my physicals and checkups from my doctors. I couldn't let any unseen illnesses go undetected. I knew of some lumps on my thyroid from the time in high school when I gave my parents a scare when these lumps were detected. My parents were frightened because cancer ran in our family. I made sure to do self-exams on my thyroid to make sure no new lumps were present. It seemed just like out of the blue when I felt an unusual larger amount of lumps connected to my thyroid. My primary doctor referred me to an endocrinologist to get these lumps biopsied. Once at the doctor, I laid my head down with my neck over a pillow so she could get the right angle, and she stuck the needle in my neck three times. The pain seemed familiar because of the time I had these lumps biopsied before but the anxiety was stronger than ever. I waited two days for the results when the doctor called to say, "Not cancerous." My joy was seconds when the doctor said it would be best to get my thyroid out because of the family history of cancer. She referred me to a surgeon. **2003—Thyroidectomy surgery**—Removal of the entire thyroid because of glandular lumps. I stayed over night in the hospital and was released after two days. When I woke, stitches and a bandage covered the bottom portion of my neck. The pain made its presence within minutes. My mother flew to my aid after surgery. She found out about a plastic surgeon that specialized in hands. I flew to Las Vegas in the next couple of weeks to see him. I loved seeing my mother again and was so excited to meet this doctor but I had little faith because all the doctors who had ever looked at my hand just told me there was no hope because any movement I would have gotten back after stroke I would have seen in the first year of recovery. After ten years I only had very little movement and spacticity had taken over my arm and hand with extreme amounts of pain because of the severe contractures. The surgeon looked at my hand and said those dreaded words, I can't help you. He did know of a neurologist that administered botox injections for the arm after stroke to relieve spasticity. My mom and I drove across town to meet this neurologist. I was hoping for the best but lived by the saying, if it's too good to be true, it usually is. I met Dr. Ginsburg and he told me of a clinical study that is for stroke patients and spasticity after stroke. The details were: I would have to get ten injections of botox in the affected arm every six weeks and at the end of the study I would have been a part of what would make botox injections suitable for FDA approval. I wanted to keep up my good deeds of making things possible for the disabled. My problem was I couldn't afford a plane ticket to Las Vegas every six weeks. My mom asked if she split the cost with me, if I could make the trips, I could. My mother has always been there for me and now she was making it possible for me to fly to Las Vegas every six weeks to get botox injections into my arm to relieve my pain from spasticity. At the end of the six weeks the botox did relieve spasticity and I helped get botox injections approved through the FDA. I grieved for the girl I once was. I had to try and separate my thoughts of what was suppose to be and develop new dreams of the girl that is to be.

CHAPTER 8

▼

("Plans I have for you,"
Declares the Lord.
Plans to give you
Hope and a future.)
Jeremiah 29:11

Life has carried on after stroke. It seems as though my emotions are on a constant cycle of ups and downs. Once again I applied for Medicare/social security and was turned down for the reason that I wasn't disabled enough. I was deeply distressed because of this. I am disabled from paralysis after stroke and I'm unemployed as a result of this. I felt I was paying the price for all of the people who dishonestly come about getting social security. I was not going to give up on something I rightfully deserved. I continued my own therapy from the notes I have taken in the past. Each time I went to outpatient therapy, I was put together with therapists that were only familiar with stroke when it first happens. I was routinely taught exercises I learned years ago from Jill. I found out the hard way that most therapists aren't familiar with post-stroke exercises. I was now forced to interview each therapist before I would make an appointment to see them. I had no training in therapy, all I knew was my body was in need of extensive **post**-stroke therapy from a therapist who could teach me new exercises, and I was going to fight to get the help my body needed. A brain injury from a stroke acts like a road block stopping the messages from getting through to the different muscles groups. If I was able to learn new exercises I could help teach my brain new pathways to teach my muscles how to work again. I had to be my body's sole caretaker because no one else was going to do it. My only source of income was unemployment. I was only allowed so many visits of therapy from the state insurance I had, and then I would be cut off. If it wasn't hard enough to be disabled so suddenly, I was forced to fight my way through the red tape of government and insurance issues to provide help for my body. When Kevin finished work on the weekends he would stay at his parents' house in Lake Tahoe so he wouldn't have to make the long drive home. I would spend my time at home doing therapy and walking Holly outside to add to my routine of therapy. Feelings of extreme loneliness invaded my every thought, not because I was physically alone but I felt alone because no one could possibly know how I felt being so young and living with paralysis after stroke. I would not force this upon my husband. I had to find the strength to carry the effects of stroke myself because I loved him too much to make him feel the way I felt daily. Kevin was always understanding of my disabilities, but until a person lives their life after stroke, they couldn't know how I feel.

One weekend I went to bed early watching television. Three days had passed, I awoke in the hospital; a nurse was asking me if I wanted to shower before I went home. I had no answer and no recollection of the last three days. I was in complete confusion as to what was happening to me. I finally saw a familiar face; Kevin walked into the room. He was coming to take me home. He explained to me, while in Lake Tahoe, he had an overwhelming feeling that he needed to come home. He raced back home. He unlocked the door and Holly was by the door which seemed odd to him as she never left my side. He called out to me with no response. Kevin ran back to our bedroom and found me hanging upside down off the bed. My mouth was frothing and I was seizing. Kevin called 911 immediately. I continued the seizures in the ambulance and at the hospital until the early hours of the morning as Kevin helplessly looked on. I was admitted into the hospital again. I had no memory of the night of seizing, times when Kevin would lay by me while he stared at the dinners I didn't eat, or lying by my side until I fell asleep and he couldn't stay any longer. Once again I was leaving the hospital. I had a relapse of seizures because after I was seizure free for three years, my last neurologist said if I passed the required tests I could get off all seizure medications. I was happy to be off any of the medications because just the co-pays of the medications were expensive. I passed all the tests but as I would find out, my body wasn't in agreement with this. I would need to take seizure medication for the rest of my life to prevent any recurring seizures. My driver's license was taken away from me for the third time. I felt like an elderly person who was trying desperately to keep their independence but losing. I had to be very diligent about taking my medications timely, getting enough rest, and surrounding myself in a stress free environment to keep the seizures away.

One year had passed when I entered the DMV to reinstate my driver's license. I accepted my paralysis but this didn't stop the grieving I felt for the girl I once was. I walked up to the next window with the necessary paperwork and doctor's script to get my license back. The woman behind the desk stared me down, looked at my wedding ring, and said, "I can't believe you are wearing that and look like that, and I look like this and I'm not wearing a wedding ring." Most people are accepting of others with disabilities but some are extremely cruel. I was sending out three resumes a month and received letters of denial every time I checked my mail. I was getting denied employment, I found out, because of all of the gaps in my work history with all of the hospital visits. I tried Medicare/social security; again and again I was turned down. In between all of the denial letters, I noticed it had been a few months since I had the botox treatments; the spasticity was getting increasingly stronger each week. The contractions in my hand and fingers were starting to make my hand curl inwards with severe pain. I would spend my nights awake trying to uncurl my fingers to relieve the pain. When I would walk my body would work as a whole so each time I would take a step, my arm would twist upwards while my fingers and hand would curl inwards. I found myself isolating myself and only going outside to walk Holly. I didn't want anyone to see me. I didn't want to have to depend on the botox injections for the rest of my life. The neurologist in Las Vegas said there were no other doctors in Reno that administered botox injections for spasticity. I refused to believe that, especially after I contributed to a study for the FDA approval for botox for arm spasticity after stroke. I started calling every neurologist in Reno. I asked if they did the botox injections or if they knew of a doctor that administered botox for spasticity. Every neurologist I called said they didn't do botox injections for spasticity and a few office staff made jokes on how I could get botox for my face down the street at the local dermatology office. I didn't laugh; I didn't think my pain was funny. On the last call before I was going to give up, I was only asking for staff management, a woman told me I could only get botox injections from one neurologist in all of Reno, at Dr. Hue's office. I called for an appointment but I had to wait a month to get in. By this point, I was getting no sleep because of the pain. Insurance denied the botox injections; they would need proof that I was disabled by stroke and that I was in need of them. I sent out letters to all of my doctors to get them all to write statement letters to state when I had my stroke and what residual problems the stroke left me with. Once I received all of the letters, I sent them off to my insurance to fight to get the botox injections I needed, and then I was approved. My only thought to get a job was that I still retained all of my hair information in my memory, and if I could reinstate my license, I could go to cosmetology school for another 600 hours or so and get a teachers license. My problem was I didn't have the use of my arm. The manager of the cosmetology school told me I could contact the ADA (Associates for the Disabled Act) for help. I started preparing for the state exam and brushing up on all things I had forgotten during the stroke. I was elated to be studying hair and I was finally getting back a part of my life that was so missed. I was happy until I got the denial letter from the ADA explaining that a hair cut was in the state exam and they were not going to take the test for me. It had been so many years since my last reinstatement; I couldn't just pay the required fee. All I could do at this point was not to give up because I loved living. Because I had been out of a job for so long, the insurance I had expired so the botox injections were going to stop soon. One day while opening up our mail, I received a letter from the social security office. I couldn't imagine what they wanted because I already knew I was denied. The letter explained that through all of the past years and applications, they had made a mistake on my case. I should have been approved years before, which would automatically make me eligible for Medicare insurance. I contacted Dr. Hue's office; they said the botox injections were approved through Medicare so I was back on the schedule every three months for the botox.

I spent most of my time indoors doing therapy; this was and is my life. I wasn't going to have my stroke and all of the depression surrounding stroke affect my marriage or the care I would give to my animals. I have now incorporated two birds with Holly to help with depression. I wanted to put a positive twist on all of the negativity that I was feeling. In **2005**, I wrote my story and submitted it to the Stroke Connection magazine, I wanted to see if my story could help someone else surviving stroke. I received a call from the editor; they wanted to use my article the following month. In my words, they constructed the following....

A New Appreciation-
May 3, 1994—For the third day I awoke with a horrible pain pounding the right side of my brain. I went to work as usual, but towards the end of the day, the pain exploded to a higher level and then sudden relief—all within a few seconds. I looked in the mirror and noticed the whole left side of my face fall. Then I fell from disorientation, weakness and loss of muscle tone on my whole left side. Some one called 9-1-1. The paramedics seemed perplexed, I assume, because of my age, 27. My blood pressure was 162/116; heart rate 83. At the trauma center in Las Vegas, a neurologist determined I'd had a massive stroke. My survival was 50/50 due to the brain swelling from the blood around my brain. When I awoke on Mothers Day, I was downgraded from CCU to ICU to a hospital stay then to rehab—2 ½ months total. My last day in the rehab hospital, my quadriceps moved by my own will. My face muscles have returned thanks to electrical stimulation (e-stem). This machine sends messages from the brain to the muscle to help the muscle remember how to work. With the help of all of my therapists, I exercised morning, noon, and evening. The movement in my leg returned, and with the aid of a cane and ankle brace, I said goodbye to my wheelchair. In 2000, I had a radical new surgery to fuse my ankle and foot bones. Now I can walk without a cane or a foot brace. May 3, 1997—Three years to the day after my stroke, I married Kevin, my soul mate. He is responsible for the

**return of my self-esteem. Soon we will celebrate our eighth year
together. I am currently enrolled in a medical research study investi-
gating spasticity after stroke. Now my arm has relaxed and I no longer
experience pain there. Because Of my stroke I have a new sense of self
and a new appreciation for faith, hope, and life.**
Renee Wines—Survivor

I walked daily as a part of my therapy; I started getting pain throughout
my right hip constantly throughout the day. I figured I was walking too
much. I went to the doctor for an X-ray on my hip. Maybe I cracked a
bone during one of my many falls. I wasn't worried until my primary doctor called me early one morning. He said I had a problem with my right
hip. I had "Avascular Necrosis". This is a disorder in which an area of
bone, my right hip, had a lack of blood supply and was dying. My doctor
had an urgent call into an orthopedic surgeon for me to see. The next
week I saw Dr. Smith. My X-ray showed him that my whole hip would
need replacing by a titanium joint for a total hip replacement. He said this
probably happened during the seizure episode I had a few months back
and a crack in the bone occurred. The bone hadn't healed correctly. I
would have a hospital stay for a few days, and I would need a walker for six
weeks afterwards until the surgery healed. I sensed nervousness come over
Dr. Smith when I explained about my stroke; I couldn't use a walker
because of the left sided paralysis. I would be forced to use a quad cane for
one hand, my right hand. A quad cane is a cane connected to four legs for
stability. I was given a list of restrictions for my body after surgery. No
bending at the hip, no crossing my legs, no baths in the bathtub, no reach-
ing, no lifting, no kneeling and more.

2006—Total Hip Replacement Surgery—Diseased bone is replaced
with a titanium joint to relieve pain. The natural bone grows into the joint
as it heals.

I awoke in the hospital again. I wasn't able to move any part of my right
hip without extreme pain. I held my urine as long as I could so I wouldn't
experience the pain of lifting my body. The very next day, a therapist
approached my room. I knew that I would have to stand. I didn't want to
but I had to pull together every ounce of strength I had ever known to

accomplish standing again and then walking through extreme pain. I sat at the edge of the hospital bed, and scooted slowly to the edge. I thought, I learned to walk once and now I would have to learn again under different circumstances. I stood on the ground for a second as the pain shot through my body. My reactions were tears and to sit down immediately, but I fought through the pain and stood up straight and made a couple of steps using a quad cane. The therapist asked if I would like to walk to the door and then come back to bed and sit. I told her that I would rather keep walking all the way down the hall to the nurse's station and back. The therapist said she had never seen a will to survive like mine, and she said the more I walked, the faster I would get better. I walked down the hall to the nurse's station and back. I couldn't wait to walk again, but for now I had to rest. My mom would be there for me, the love and bond we had made her my willing caretaker. She flew down to take care of me while I healed.

Every chance I got I was outside walking with my mom or with Holly until I was strong enough to walk alone. I started substituting walks for pain medication. I am forced to stay out of work because now that I fought to get Social Security and Medicare, it would be a contradiction to work and they would take my social security away. I was getting botox injections every three months, ten needles each time, up and down my left arm. I had to prove my disability to Medicare before each botox treatment, until I wrote a stern letter to them to start recognizing that I was disabled because of stroke. I didn't and wouldn't always have to prove my disability. The whole process was exhausting and I did not want to have to depend on botox injections for the rest of my life so I researched an orthopedic surgeon for my hand; I was refereed to Dr. Christiansen. I still had to monitor anything that popped up on or in my body; I noticed a small clear/reddish lump on my nose. I went to my primary doctor right away to see if this lump, that never seemed to go away, was okay. He assured me it was fine and I was probably overreacting. In my gut, I still didn't feel this was normal. I made an appointment to see a dermatologist for a second opinion. I couldn't take the chance with my family history of cancer. The doctor plunged a needle into my nose, both my eyes watered and I could hardly breathe through the pain and tears. The biopsy came back as skin cancer.

2007—Moh's skin cancer surgery—Moh's is a technique to ensure every bit of cancer is removed. In this procedure the patient has to be awake and given needles to numb the area while cutting is taking place. The doctor sat me in the chair while she injected my nose four times. The pain was excruciating and it seemed as though every nerve in my body was firing at once. The doctor sliced a section away and looked at the section she cut under the microscope. I waited in the waiting area with other skin cancer surgery patients. We each had a bandage on a different area of the face. Ear, chin, forehead, and me, the nose. We were all waiting for the doctor to say you're done and we got all the cancer. Just then, the doctor's aide called my name. She said we didn't get it all, we have to cut more. My heart sunk as I walked back into the surgery room. My finger tips dug into the arm chair while the doctor stuck another four needles into my nose. I repeated this stage three more times during the day while the doctor struggled to get all the cancer that was growing into fingered lines through my nose. I was relieved when finally the doctor said they got it all and I could go across the street to the plastic surgeons office for repair of the hole in my nose. I was at the point of pure exhaustion as I slumped into the waiting doctor's chair. The doctor took the bandage off and touched the area with a Q-tip. I nearly came off the chair from the pain that filled my body. The doctor said that I should look at the area after surgery. I didn't want to; I knew it was bad because the last doctor had been cutting on my nose from 9AM until 4:30 PM. The doctor handed me the mirror. I lifted it up to my face, and I felt my heart crying silent tears that I had come to know well. The hole in my nose was a dime shape and bloodied. The pain that radiated from it I couldn't stand any longer, so the doctor thought it was best to repair the hole a different day after I rested.

2007-Plastic surgery Repair—Delicately repairing the area to cover the hole in my nose. A month later I made plans for my next surgery. Dr. Christiansen was the best hand surgeon in Reno, Nevada.

2007, Wrist/Finger tendon lengthening surgery—Lengthening the shortened tendons from paralysis, that should automatically lengthen and shorten with normal movement.

This surgery was done to eliminate the pain and the botox injections every three months. The surgery was a day surgery and the pain I was getting prior to surgery was more severe than the recovery after surgery. Dr. Christiansen told me prior to surgery that my thumb was so contracted that I might have to have a second surgery.

2007-Thumb tendon lengthening/muscle cutting/pinning surgery—Tendon lengthening and muscle would need to be cut in the web of the thumb to release the contraction and pinning to help with healing in a normal placement.

Dr. Christiansen told me that there could be a third surgery to fuse the thumb. After the surgery had healed, the surgery worked in the fact that my fingers and thumb can close in correlation with each other, but because the brain injury is so massive, extension of the fingers and thumb is not possible. I have good and bad days following stroke and paralysis. The secret to my survival is not to let the negativity take root and try to turn negatives into positives whenever possible. I will eternally be grateful for the second chance at life God has given me and for the love of my husband Kevin, my soul mate. I'm convinced it would have been a love I would have never known.

EPILOGUE

$\blacktriangledown$

("Carve a tunnel of hope through the dark
Mountain of disappointment.")
Martin Luther King Jr.

Have faith in your body's ability to heal itself. In time healing does take place. The extent and pace of recovery from stroke and brain injury varies between survivors. The majority of stroke survivors show signs of recovery within the first six months to one year post-stroke. Healthy brain cells take over the functions of damaged brain cells known as brain plasticity. Some survivors show great improvement following stroke, through physical, occupational, and speech therapy for up to as far out as ten years post-stroke. I am thirteen years post-stroke and see small signs with the aide of advanced surgeries. I have built my life around my disability. I can't plan for the unknown but I'm compelled to do so in my everyday life. I have to know ahead of time what most would not have a second thought about. I have to schedule doctor's appointments and plan my life six months in advance because doctors book up so quickly. I have to take my shower and wash my hair separate from each other because of the severe nerve discomfort I feel while in the shower. I take my shower sitting in a chair, dry myself and get dressed, and then wash my hair in the sink. I have to stay on top of my doctors to monitor my blood monthly so my medications don't affect my liver. I have to remind my doctors to issue new prescriptions for therapy. I have to fight insurance companies to approve therapy. Some doctors and most insurance companies feel that all therapy can be done at home; this is true to a point. I plan my days around therapy, mornings for occupational, evenings for physical therapy, and all throughout the day I take four to five short walks with my dog Holly. I interview any new therapists related to my case to make sure I'm getting taught the right exercises for post-stroke. I have to prove my disability to any organizations that are funded for the disabled. I have to write lists for everything because of memory loss. Birthday, Anniversary and Christmas gifts need to be purchased months before the actual event so I don't forget. I have to plan my meals a day in advance to make sure I will be able to both, open a jar and cut anything using the one handed props I have for cutting. I deal with stroke and paralysis by approaching life as it comes with a good attitude. What I want other stroke survivors to realize is that life doesn't end because of stroke and paralysis but in some ways it begins. In the event of stroke, I have come to know life in a different way. It's precious and I don't take it for granted. Flowers are vibrant in color, birds whistling bring peace and harmony throughout my body, and the love of my spouse and animals brings a joy that lives deep within my soul. I tell my story from my heart to help other stroke survivors in their journey of recovery in hopes to lend some comfort that life doesn't end there. My hope is to hold out for a cure for stroke and I have faith that some day it will come.

About the Author

Born in St. Petersburg, Florida, raised in Las Vegas, Nevada. After high school, I modeled in conventions while building a career in cosmetology.

Before, during, and after my illness, I attended different colleges, I took classes in diverse subjects to stay well educated. I live in Reno, Nevada with my husband of ten years and my three animals, a dog and two birds. My interests are reading, scrap-booking, home-making, & animal care.

978-0-595-47223-9
0-595-47223-0

Made in the USA
Lexington, KY
19 April 2011